Suppo. _ _ _.
Do You Really Need Spine Surgery?

"All these doctors said their surgeries would have over an 80 percent chance of success, but surgery did nothing but cause more pain. Your work has helped me more than ANY treatment I ever received from over the 30 physicians I went to. I would like to explain how much I have improved both mentally and physically in the last year since I started applying your concepts and Dr. Sarno's concepts. I went back to full duty last October and I'm working in a busy area. I work out all the time doing intense cardio three days a week and weight lifting. I feel great and don't take any medication. I started doing hobbies such as wood working and fishing again. I'm playing with my children instead of lying on the couch all day half high on Oxycodone. To put it simply, I have my life back. I just wish I knew about all this years ago."
   —John D., Fire Captain

"Dr. Hanscom's work has become a central component in how we manage our patients with chronic lower back pain. His latest book will be essential for educating patients about their options regarding spine surgery. I believe this book should be recommended to anyone who is considering surgery. The book is well organized and accessible for both patients and clinicians. Every rehabilitation specialist, including chiropractors, acupuncturists, and physical therapists, should have this book as a resource for their clients and themselves!"
   —Stuart Eivers, DPT, OCS, FAAOMPT

"Dr. Hanscom provides patients and their health care providers the information needed to make a rational choice regarding when to undergo spinal surgery. He also outlines the treatment and work that is required prior to any spine surgery. This book is also a resource for primary care physicians who refer their patients to spine surgeons. The information, along with references, will allow them to support their patients and hold the surgeons accountable for their surgical recommendations, based on documented best practices."
   —Joel Konikow, MD

"David Hanscom's recent book, *Do You Really Need Spine Surgery?* is a most necessary addition to the spine treatment lexicon. His writing is amazingly clear, and he systematically analyzes the thought processes necessary for correct surgical decision making. It is destined to become required reading both for patients and definitely for their doctors."
   —David Cassius, MD, Physical Medicine and Rehab,
   Pain Medicine

"I have been living with chronic pain since 1993 and have had ten operations, resulting in my entire lumbar spine being fused. Dr. Hanscom performed the last of my surgeries. I feel that if I had met him sooner, the last twenty years would have been much different. I am so grateful for the knowledge I have gained working with him. I always tell people how he truly gave me back my life."
   —Cheryl Hungate, former patient

"I am a retired neurosurgeon who performed spine surgery for many years. I then moved on to manage chronic pain and opioid addiction. I have read hundreds of chronic pain books and thousands of scientific articles.

"I also have disabling chronic pain in my feet. I purchased Dr. Hanscom's first amazing book. *Back in Control: A Surgeon's Roadmap Out of Chronic Pain*, and can say without reservation that this is the best chronic pain book that I have ever read. I recommend that every person with chronic pain get this book and read it repeatedly. Although I have treated chronic pain for decades, I did not have the insight to institute my treatment plans in such an easy to do format. He advises all of us to become our own healers. My hope is to also cure myself of my chronic pain! Thank you Dr. Hanscom for your valuable contribution to all the legions of people with chronic pain."
   — Retired neurosurgeon

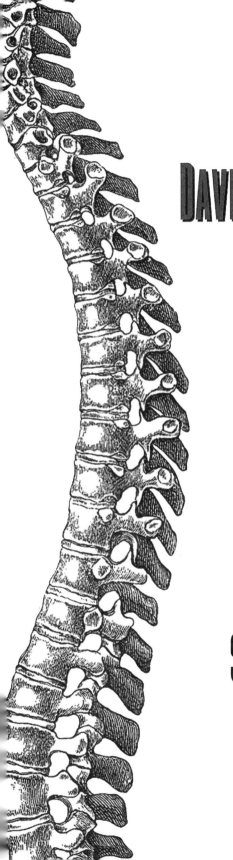

DAVID HANSCOM, M.D.

DO
YOU
REALLY
NEED
SPINE
SURGERY?

*Take Control
with a Surgeon's Advice*

Do You Really Need Spine Surgery?

Copyright © 2019 by David Hanscom, MD

Published by Vertus Press
617 Kenwyn Rd
Oakland, CA 94610

ISBN: 978-0988272965
eISBN: 978-0988272910

Library of Congress Number 2019912023

Printed in the United States of America

Interior Layout: Marcia Breece
Cover Design: James Rothbart
eBook: Marcia Breece

While all of the patient stories described in this book are based on true experiences, all of the names are pseudonyms, and some situations have been changed slightly for educational purposes and to protect each individual's privacy.

The information in this book is not offered, nor should it be used to treat or diagnose any particular disease or any particular patient. Neither the author nor the publisher is engaged in rendering professional advice or services to the individual reader.

This book is dedicated to my patients
who have connected with their capacity to heal
in the face of what seemed like insurmountable odds.

The essence of the solution for chronic pain is connecting to your own capacity to heal.

CONTENTS

FOREWORD

The story you are about to read is the first of three histories I am presenting to illustrate why I am writing this book. It represents a common scenario where spine surgery is recommended or performed on anatomy that is not a source of pain. In such cases, surgery not only is ineffective, but often it makes patients worse.

Sachit Egan

"You can choose to leave my office today without scheduling your surgery, but you will regret it. Patients with your spinal anatomy will inevitably break down, and the pain will be debilitating. I guarantee that you'll come back to me within three years, and you'll *beg* me for surgery."

I stared at the doctor, totally dumbfounded. I'd spent the past eighteen months exploring options for relieving the intense back pain that had erupted in my early twenties. After the typical non-invasive treatments (epidural injections, physical therapy, chiropractic care) hadn't produced lasting results, I decided that surgery was the next logical step. In many ways, it also felt like my last hope.

I had grown up a bookworm, spending much of my childhood indoors and pouring myself into books and video games. I remember complaining endlessly one middle school day when my family dragged me off the couch for a trip to Muir Woods. However, my outlook changed following an overnight hike of Yosemite's Half Dome during my freshman year of college. As we watched the sun rise over the distant peaks, I decided to refocus my life on spending time outdoors.

I quickly picked up rock climbing, trail running, and backpacking, and I started an outdoor recreation program at my university. I maintained an intense exercise regimen to build strength and endurance for these activities, taking this training as seriously as I did my studies. After graduating, I moved to Alaska and began leading river rafting and backpacking trips near Denali

National Park. Indeed, I had come to view being an outdoorsman as a key component of my identity.

Sadly, things soon changed again—this time for the worse: One afternoon, while picking up a heavy box of equipment, I felt a snap in my lower back. Within days, I found myself hunched over with nerve-wrenching pain in my back and right leg. On my twenty-third birthday, I was unable to walk two blocks from my car to a restaurant. As I sat on the sidewalk that afternoon, I distinctly remember thinking to myself: Will I ever be able to climb Half Dome again?

Eighteen months of non-invasive treatments did yield one positive result: A skilled chiropractor was able to fully resolve my leg pain. However, the crippling back pain still remained. At this point, I felt the hopelessness that is all too common among those afflicted with chronic back pain

Desperate to return to my previous form, I felt surgery looming as the only remaining option. Within weeks of my twenty-third birthday, I had appointments lined up with three of the top spine surgeons in the Bay Area. To my surprise, their advice was identical: "Have surgery *now*. Do not pass GO, do not collect $200... just have surgery as soon as possible."

Given the magnitude of the procedures they proposed (multi-level fusions, potentially with artificial disc replacements), one of them (the chief of spine surgery at a name-brand hospital) remarkably pushed to schedule surgery for the following week. In hindsight, I'm amazed that I agreed to this proposal—we were discussing a wholly life-altering procedure, and we didn't even allow for research or preparation time.

With surgery scheduled just days away, I received a tremendous stroke of good fortune: a trusted friend recommended Dr. Hanscom's first book to me (*Back in Control*). I picked it up and pored over it throughout the weekend. With newfound hope, I canceled my surgery and opted to call Dr. Hanscom's office in Washington. A few weeks later, I made the trip to Seattle to visit him in person. I'll never forget his first words upon entering the examination room: "You shouldn't even be considering surgery. Based on your anatomy, you're simply not a candidate. It's a failure of our medical system that anyone would even recommend surgery to you."

After Dr. Hanscom convinced me to rule out surgery, I admit it took some time to discern my next steps. Dr. Hanscom had assured me that my pain wasn't related to anatomy or injuries in my spine. As such, I felt I had nothing to lose by carefully attempting to reintroduce my old hobbies into my life. I began with light weightlifting and aerobic exercise, which I ramped up over time. Eventually I introduced hiking, then backpacking, and then rock climbing. Six years later, I'm in the best shape of my life: I make an annual trip to Yosemite and Half Dome, and I'm happy to say I've never reconsidered surgery. I'll always be grateful that I met Dr. Hanscom during a scary time in my life, and that I didn't follow through with spine surgery when I was twenty-three.

—Sachit Egan, 2019

This second story is written by Mark Owens, the gentleman who wrote the Foreword to my book, *Back in Control: A Surgeon's Roadmap Out of Chronic Pain.* After breaking his back in a horse riding accident and undergoing an appropriate surgery to stabilize his spine, Mark developed chronic back pain. A second operation on a degenerated disc just below his fusion was not indicated, and it worsened his condition. Years later, about to undergo a twelve-hour fusion from his neck to his pelvis, Mark saw me for one final opinion. With a structured, non-surgical approach to his pain, he avoided surgery and is now fully active without pain.

Dr. Mark Owens is a remarkable person in many ways. He is an environmental scientist who went to Africa with his new wife, Delia, with the intention of researching and conserving wildlife. He and Delia spent twenty-three years there, researching Kalahari Desert wildlife and setting up conservation programs for elephants and human communities in the Rift Valley of Zambia. Their model community conservation programs saved tens of thousands of elephants while raising the living standards of rural communities all over northeast Zambia. After more than thirty years the Owens legacy continues as the North Luangwa Community Conservation Project, still a viable entity. Their adventures are chronicled in their three best-selling books, *Cry of the Kalahari (Owens), The Eye of The Elephant,* and *Secrets of The Savanna.*

Not everyone was supportive of his efforts. Mark and his wife had twenty-four hours to flee Africa when he learned of a third assassination attempt by the government-sponsored ivory poachers. They settled in Idaho, where they set up a large nature reserve to protect grizzly bears and wolves. It was in the mountains of Idaho, while Mark was surveying the area for grizzlies, that his horse threw him, crushing his spine and chest. He almost died of exposure while waiting for rescue on the mountain, but fortunately he was not paralyzed. An emergency surgery to stabilize his thoracic spine was successful. Normally, he would have been pain-free and fully functional within three to four months, but he developed chronic, debilitating pain.

Dr. Owens is one of the toughest human beings I have ever met. How could this happen? You will learn in this book how injuries develop into chronic pain.

Following is Mark's story, in his own words, of his journey out of crippling pain. It begins on the mountain, at the moment of his rescue, when he at last realized he wasn't going to freeze to death. He had just spent all night on the cold ground, severely injured, waiting for his riding partner to return with help.

Mark Owens

The Libby Search and Rescue arrived with a doctor who immediately injected me with Fentanyl, wrapped me in a foil blanket, and stuffed me into a bivvy bag filled with hot water bottles. Then the team strapped me to a stretcher and began carrying me up the pitch-black trail to a high alpine meadow, where a helicopter met us at sunrise and flew me to the Kalispell, Montana Regional hospital. There a surgeon installed a foot-long ladder of steel in my back, re-inflated my collapsed lung and sent me home to recover. I will always remember his parting words, "From now on, Mark, your life will be all about pain control." But I was optimistic: I knew I could do better than that.

And yet, by 2012, six years after my accident, I again had so much pain in my lower back that I had another surgery to fuse L2 and L3. I had barely recovered from that when, driving with too little sleep and

By the spring of 2013, my legs were collapsing under me, I was holding onto furniture to keep from falling, and my pain levels were constantly between eight and ten. I began looking for another surgeon who could release me from this hell, and I found one in eastern Washington who explained that he had been a General Motors auto engineer before going to medical school.

"Your back has seen too much trauma," he said. "You really don't have any good options, and most of them would not relieve you of your pain or improve your range of motion. The only hope for you is what I call the Blue Plate Special." He went on to explain a two-day surgery during which he and another surgeon would filet me like a salmon, incising me from my clavicle to my pelvis in order to remove the titanium steel hardware that was buried in the straight, stiff fusion mass that spanned from the 8th thoracic to the second lumbar vertebra. After breaking my spine through the fusion in two places, they would then replace the existing construct with a longer, more curved one that would better conform to the natural curvature of my original spine. Finally, they would remove calcium deposits, causing stenosis in my spinal canal, and extend the fusion to my pelvis. Most of my spine would become one solid piece of bone and hardware.

He presented all of this with what seemed to me to be fairly unrestrained glee, confidence bordering on over-confidence, and an air of certitude that defied his words when he said, "This will be quite a complicated surgery with a fair amount of risk and a long recovery; but frankly, any more conservative surgical options are bound to fail, leaving you worse off than you are now."

This wasn't the first time a surgeon had recommended this type of radical operation to me: Before my fusion in 2012, another doctor had proposed something similar. Still, to hear it again was tough. At that point my mood could best be described as somber; his words were like lead weights pulling my head under water for the last time. He was so good at selling this surgery, however, that I felt strongly inclined to sign up for it right there and then, especially when he said that he could schedule the procedure within six weeks of that date. But in the end I left, telling him I'd have to think it over.

I walked out with the friend who was with me and before we even got to the parking lot, it hit me. I couldn't just go by this

I walked out with the friend who was with me and before we even got to the parking lot, it hit me. I couldn't just go by this doctor's word for such a drastic procedure. I turned to my friend and said, "What if this is more about ego than what would be good for me? I need another opinion."

Two days later we entered the office of Dr. David Hanscom in Seattle. Seconds after coming through the door he announced: "I've looked at the images of your back and I'm afraid I cannot recommend surgery for you. I don't see a one-to-one correspondence between any dysfunction in your spine and the pain you are experiencing."

My mouth fell open in shock. Dr. Hanscom went on to explain that only about 20 – 30% of fusion surgeries for low back pain are successful in relieving back pain, meaning that 70 – 80% are not. Furthermore, many of these surgeries leave patients worse off than they were before.

My Assessment

Mark's situation was actually straightforward based on the medical literature. He had three levels of disc degeneration below his prior fusion, which ran from his 8th thoracic vertebrae to the 3rd lumbar vertebrae. There is no evidence that degeneration is a source of chronic back pain (Boden). I felt not a flicker of inclination that his spine needed further surgery. I had already seen hundreds of patients free themselves from chronic pain, in ways similar to those that helped me return to a normal life during my own bout with debilitating chronic pain. I had quit performing fusions for back pain over twenty years earlier, when I saw the data that showed a success rate of less than 30%, two years after surgery (Franklin, Carragee). For a long time, I had nothing to offer my patients, but I knew I wasn't going to put them through this level of surgery with such a low chance of a successful outcome.

Mark's Response

I felt strangely deflated and disoriented—as though I'd been given bad news, not good. "But what am I supposed to do? I'm not imagining this pain, and my legs are collapsing." Like so many other chronic back-pain sufferers, I could feel myself growing desperate to be sliced and diced because I had been programmed by ten different surgeons to believe that it was my only option.

"I think you're suffering from a chronically stressed nervous system, which causes persistent elevation of your survival hormones such as cortisol, adrenaline and histamine. This situation affects every cell and organ in your body and translates into over thirty physical symptoms. One experiences more pain from increased speed of nerve conduction (Chen). Additionally, your brain memorizes the pain, similar to riding a bicycle, and you are stuck with it. You can't unlearn it. So, your brain is creating its own endogenous pain stimuli, rather like "phantom limb syndrome," registering pain even though the offending appendage has been removed." David went on to explain that research in neuroscience has confirmed that after about three months, chronic pain sufferers' brains rewire themselves with neural connections to newly developed brain centers that generate their own pain signals. These signals are independent of any dysfunction in the body below the victim's head (Hashmi).

I was candid with the doctor: I wasn't convinced. "To be honest, this sounds a little like snake oil to me," I said.

"Well, you can choose to go under the knife again with all of its associated risks and limitations, or you can read my book and learn about using simple techniques that even a grade-schooler can master, and maybe rid yourself of your chronic pain forever. You can start right away with "expressive writing." You simply spend fifteen to thirty minutes in the morning and again at night, writing down, in longhand, any thought that comes into your head. After you've written out each one in graphic and descriptive language, you immediately tear it up."

My friend and I left David's office feeling that this was too good to be true, but I also resolved to try this literature-based approach to pain control before submitting to radical surgery (Baikie).

We drove south along the coast from Seattle, found a motel for the night, and I immediately tried my hand at expressive writing. I was quite sure it would never work for me. David had explained that different types of expressive writing, as well as other techniques used in his program, are supported by a growing body of peer-reviewed scientific research, but I had not yet seen this work. As a scientist, I am skeptical by nature. Nonetheless, at that point I was willing to give anything a try.

The next morning when I awoke, I noticed that my lower back hadn't greeted me with a shot of pain before I even moved my legs to get up from bed, something that had occurred for years.

"No way; this cannot be," I said to myself as I stretched out my legs, fully expecting the usual lightning bolt of pain. But all I felt was a comparatively mild discomfort. I stood up and walked to the bathroom. Yes, it hurt as I walked, but nothing like it had since my accident in 2006. Still, I refused to credit the writing I had done.

We drove on into Oregon that day, and by late afternoon we found ourselves lying on a nearly deserted beach with our heads on a chunk of driftwood, watching gulls wheeling overhead as the surf caressed our feet.

"I am afraid to believe this," I said to my friend, "but for the very first time in nine years I am virtually pain-free—and happy. It's as if a veil of agony has lifted from my face and I can see the world clearly again." I estimated that in less than two days I had somehow gotten rid of about 80% of my chronic pain.

It took me a while to trust this sudden release from the hell of chronic pain, but today, over five years later, I go as much as an entire week at a stretch without needing to take any analgesics at all, not even Tylenol. Gradually my world has expanded again, and as I write this, I am planning a horseback ride back up the Cedar Creek trail where I nearly died thirteen years ago. It has become a regular pilgrimage for me, I think, because I still cannot fully comprehend how I managed to escape the grip of soul-destroying chronic pain that so many others are enduring—many of them needlessly. If you are one of them, read on: This book will save your life (Hanscom). I know, because it surely saved mine.

I am grateful that I was able to avoid such a large operation that had such a low chance of success and a high complication rate. I shudder to think how my life may have turned out had I proceeded with surgery. But it is upsetting to me that this option was even recommended to me when the solutions were so simple and accessible. This was a largely self-directed process. I essentially lost nine years of a productive and enjoyable life, and it had a devastating effect on my personal life. It could have been so different, and I am still dealing with the aftermath of it all.

Although I appeared to be the "perfect patient" to my doctors, they didn't take the time to get to know me. I handle stress well, but I was wearing down. My nervous system was extremely sensitized, as I had a lot going on in my life at the time my back was first broken. I clearly did not need the second operation, which dramatically worsened my pain. I now know what the research confirms: that performing any type of surgery in the presence of untreated chronic pain often worsens it (Perkins). To recover from chronic, crippling pain within a couple of months is mind-boggling. Please read this book carefully before making any surgical decisions that will affect your entire quality of life.

We are on the cusp of a revolution in treating chronic pain, whether it is emotional or physical. Dr. David Hanscom and his colleagues in this pioneering effort are risking a great deal and sacrificing much to lead the charge against the profit-oriented medical establishment in promoting a treatment that costs nothing more than a little time, commitment, and the price of a notebook and a pencil. Oh yes, and the suspension of disbelief.

David and his cohorts are truly modern day heroes in this struggle.

—Mark Owens, 2019

This final story illustrates how failed and non-indicated surgery can destroy a life. It is an increasingly frequent occurrence and the reason I retired from my complex spine surgery practice to do what I can to slow the alarming tide of aggressive spine surgery.

Patricia

I met Patricia in my office twenty-five years after she injured her lower back. She was now in her mid-sixties, wheelchair-bound, and unable to stay awake because of several hundred milligrams of morphine every day in addition to her Morphine pain pump. She was slumped over and barely could whisper, "I want my back fixed."

When I looked at Patricia's x-rays I was taken aback at what I saw: A two-level fusion at the lowest levels of her spine (lumbar 4 – 5 and L5-sacral 1), performed in an effort to relieve chronic low back pain (LBP). She continued to have the pain, though; and about a year later another fusion was performed at the next higher level, between her 3rd and 4th lumbar vertebrae. Not only did this one fail to help her pain; her spine subsequently broke above the fusion so that, when she stood up, her chest was parallel with the floor.

After that, Patricia bounced around the medical system for over twenty years, during which her spine collapsed into the shape of a pretzel, causing her to lose over seven inches of height. Her waistline totally disappeared. Her coping mechanism consisted of high doses of narcotics and smoking two packs of cigarettes a day. The situation made my decision simple: "No." There was no way she could tolerate the twelve hours of surgery needed to correct her spine. I gave her a copy of my book and told her to read it, then come back and talk in a couple of weeks. I had no expectations of seeing her again, especially after reading my book.

Two weeks later, she returned and said, "I read your book and I want surgery." Then I sat down with her again to hear her out and listen more carefully. I said I would consider doing reconstructive surgery, but she would have to prepare for it. The first step was to stop smoking. Few people can stop a two-pack-a-day habit, and once more I thought this would be the end of her visits. Although I hoped to see her back in a couple of weeks, she disappeared for eight months.

When Patricia finally returned once more, she had quit smoking. She repeated, "I want the surgery." Obviously she was serious, and she had already beaten the odds. We spent another three months stabilizing her medications, working on her nutrition, and mobilizing her outside the wheelchair as best as she could. She underwent fourteen hours of surgery in two sessions about ten days apart. We did it. She could stand up almost straight. Six months later she was upright, out of her wheelchair and using a cane, and off all medications, with minimal pain. She kicked out her husband and went back to school. I was shocked.

Patricia's miraculous recovery reinforced several of my beliefs, the first being that anyone can heal. I have never seen anyone in worse mental and physical shape and had written her off the day I met her. Second, I had long felt that humans were meant to thrive and would take the opportunity if given even the smallest chance. But some people have convinced themselves that they cannot heal and there is nothing I can do to change their trajectory if that is their choice. The main, maybe only obstacle to healing is openness to change and learning. Third, I can't tell what a person is capable of without working with them for a while.

I finally said to Patricia one day, "No one makes changes like this! You were angry, wheelchair-bound and addicted to drugs. What happened?" Her reply was simple. "I wanted to keep being a grandmother to my five year-old granddaughter."

The essence of healing is connecting to your own capacity to heal. Patricia found it.

So, in Patricia's eyes, I was a hero. I worked with her, performed major surgery, and got her out of the wheelchair and on her way to a better life. But I didn't see it that way. I regretted that I didn't meet her before she had undergone any spine surgery. She would have done well with just a solid rehab program. Instead, she had her prime of life taken from her, with a profound effect on her family. The original surgery that led to the collapse of her spine should not have been done. It is sad that the medical profession even considered surgery as an option in her case, with no data to support it.

These three stories are among hundreds of examples I have encountered, of lives ruined by ill-advised spine surgery. I am not against surgery. I am in favor of surgery when it is directed at a specific, clearly identifiable source of trouble. But even then, surgery is not the whole answer. By actively addressing *all* the factors that affect outcomes, you can make the correct choice, direct your own rehabilitation, and move on to a rich and full life.

INTRODUCTION

FROM THE DAY I ENTERED MEDICAL SCHOOL, I wanted to be an orthopedic surgeon. In 1985 I emerged from my residency and fellowship on fire, ready to solve the world's spine problems. I freely prescribed and energetically performed many spine fusions for low back pain (creating a bony bridge across vertebral segments), convinced that I was the hero freeing my patients from their misery. If I couldn't find an anatomical abnormality I could operate on, I felt guilty and helpless.

However, over time, I started observing unexplained inconsistencies in the outcomes of my procedures. Some patients didn't do as well as expected, in spite of having undergone the same, technically well-performed operation. Others felt even worse than before the surgery. I redoubled my efforts to make better decisions as to whether a person should undergo surgery, and I gave more consideration to non-operative options. I noticed some improvement— but from my perspective, not enough. I expected an operation of this magnitude to have a success rate of over 90%, and so did most of my patients. When their expectations went unmet, dealing with their dashed hopes began to wear me down.

In 1993, a study of Workers' Compensation patients in Washington State (where I worked) revealed that the success rate for lumbar spine fusions was only 15 – 25% (Franklin). Shocked, I immediately stopped performing fusions for low back pain. Even though I had no alternatives (yet), I knew this procedure wasn't a viable option.

During this time, I myself plunged into an abyss of intense chronic pain and unrelenting anxiety that many would describe as "burnout." Up to that point, I had been a fearless, top-level surgeon with a "bring it on" attitude regardless of my stress level; anxiety had been a total stranger to me. Nonetheless, by sheer willpower, I not only continued to work, but honed my skills throughout my ordeal; and somehow, after living in that hell for fifteen years, I managed to escape, understanding neither how I descended into it nor emerged from it, but with a greater appreciation for what my patients with chronic pain were going through.

Eight years after regaining control of my well being, I heard a lecture by Dr. Howard Schubiner, a pain specialist and author of the book Unlearn Your Pain. Dr. Schubiner provided a crucial piece to the puzzle by introducing me to the connection between stress and pain. He explained that chronic stress created sustained levels of survival hormones, affecting every cell in the body and causing over thirty physical and mental symptoms. I had experienced seventeen of them during my time in the "abyss." Suddenly my whole journey made sense.

I wondered why we spine surgeons weren't applying these findings in our practices, instead of rushing patients into the operating room. After all, the outcomes of spine surgery were far from 100% predictable; complications could be catastrophic; and the costs were exorbitant. Why, then, weren't we looking for ways to avoid surgery if we could? Although by this time my enthusiasm for surgical solutions had waned, I continued to watch a steady stream of other surgeon's patients go under the knife, convinced they needed surgery. Too often the operation either failed to provide relief or made matters worse, leading to more surgeries and more problems. I often heard post-operative laments such as, "If only I had known how dangerous this surgery was and what the outcome was going to be, I would have chosen against it" and "I'm a lot worse off now than I was before." We were not only failing to treat chronic pain; in many cases, we were escalating it. Every week, I would see several referrals, patients who had undergone unnecessary or inappropriate surgery on either minimal pathologies or normally aging spines. Many of them had complications that worsened their conditions, and I would do my best to salvage their backs, with or without more surgery.

All spine surgeons—regardless of skill level—will occasionally experience intra-operative and postoperative complications in their patients. I saw patients referred to me (as well as some of my own) with complications severe enough to require a brutal number of additional spine surgeries, frequently in quick succession. For example:

- Seven surgeries in ten years
- Eight operations in twelve years

- Thirteen surgeries in four years

- Fifteen surgeries in two years

- Twenty-nine operations in twenty years

The common thread running through most of these disastrous histories was that either the first surgery wasn't necessary, or the problem could have been addressed with a much smaller operation.

At the same time, I saw dozens of other patients with severe spine abnormalities who avoided surgery altogether because their pain had subsided on its own. Their doctor had taken the time to sit and talk with them, to ask them about their lives. If they were going through rough times, they were asked to first try a few exercises, which included reducing stress, improving sleep, and learning about chronic pain. It was hard to believe at first, but I saw it with my own eyes—as these were my patients. They had reduced their pain enough to opt out of surgery.

Learning from my patients' experiences, I published my first edition of *Back in Control: A Spine Surgeon's Roadmap Out of Chronic Pain* (Hanscom, 2012). As I continued to learn what did and didn't work for people with chronic back pain, I became aware of the depth of neuroscience research documenting the effects of human consciousness on the perception of pain. A few years later I published the second edition of *Back in Control,* which was more concise and research-based (Hanscom, 2016). I combined the new edition with a website, www.backincontrol.com, which houses the action plan of the book and an ever-expanding trove of supplementary material.

I witnessed hundreds of patients free themselves of pain, usually without surgery. Not only did their health improve; they often lifted their quality of life to a level they had never known before. Sharing my patients' healing journeys has been the most rewarding part of my career.

Still, when I thought of all the patients unnecessarily harmed with aggressive interventions, it weighed heavily on me. One day I met a young gentleman who had undergone a spine fusion for a problem that did not even call for surgery and was paralyzed as a result of the procedure. That was it for me. I made the decision then and there to quit my surgical practice and confront the juggernaut of aggressive spine surgery.

I am not against spine surgery. But I am strongly opposed to undergoing the risks of a major operation when the diagnosis is unclear and the outcome is unpredictable. Inasmuch as every spine surgery alters the spine, it causes some degree of permanent damage. Therefore, unless there is a distinct, identifiable problem that is correctable by a procedure, surgery should not even be considered as a treatment option.

That is why I wrote this book. In it I clearly lay out everything you need to know in order to make an informed decision about spine surgery, in partnership with your doctor. Where the stakes are so high—and take it from me, they are—you deserve to know when surgery will help and when it won't; what risks you face; what alternatives are open to you, and a great deal of other pivotal information. Armed with this knowledge, you may discover that you really do not need—nor should you have—spine surgery.

SECTION 1:
KNOW YOUR CONDITION

CHAPTER 1

The Treatment Grid

MANY PATIENTS AND HEALTH CARE PROVIDERS consider surgery the definitive solution for almost any spinal disorder after other treatments have failed. However, just because no other treatments worked doesn't mean you should head for the operating room. The Treatment Grid provides a framework for you to make the correct choices.

The key to making the right decision about spine surgery is to understand all aspects of your condition. The following two questions are pivotal:

- What is the source of my pain?

- What is the state of my nervous system?

The Source of Your Pain

When we can see an abnormality on an imaging study (such as an x-ray, CAT scan, or MRI), and your pain is symptomatic of that abnormality, we call this a structural source of pain. It is only under these circumstances that surgery should be performed. When there is no evidence of an abnormality on an imaging test, or when the symptoms do not match an observed abnormality, we call it a non-structural source of pain.

Now, here's the challenge. Usually the source of pain *cannot* be identified on an imaging test. Most pain arises from irritation and inflammation of soft tissue surrounding and supporting your skeletal system. Since there are over a million pain receptors in each square inch of these soft tissues, the discomfort is often quite severe. As you continue to move and re-irritate these areas, your pain continues. After around three months, your nervous system memorizes the pain impulses and moves them to a different part of the brain—the part that processes emotions (Hashmi). Once pain is centered in the emotional area of the brain, intense feelings such as anger and sadness can trigger, amplify, or even create sensations of pain even where there is no physical cause, often after the injury has long healed.

The Status of your Nervous System

Your stress level has a direct effect on your perception of pain. When you are mentally, verbally or physically threatened, your survival instinct takes over. Your body quickly cranks out "stress chemicals" such as adrenaline, cortisol and histamines, which ramp up your nerve conduction rates and amplify your senses. The mere thought of a threat can create a physiological fight-or-flight response, even when there is no immediate danger. I call a nervous system in this state "hyper-vigilant" or "fired up."

Any circumstance that you perceive as threatening will create a hyper-vigilant nervous system. Such circumstances can include problems with finances, relationships, your living space, work environment, chronic illness, being in the disability system, and chronic pain. Even unpleasant repetitive thoughts (URTs) impact our nervous systems, so we are all subject to hyper-vigilant nervous systems to some extent (Eisenberger).

Unless we understand and accept this aspect of the human condition and implement effective strategies to process our thoughts, our bodies will be constantly bombarded with survival hormones, negatively affecting our general health and pain thresholds. A large research paper out of Scandinavia, involving a registry of over 300,000 people, demonstrated a direct link between chronic stress and autoimmune disorders such as Crohn's disease, ulcerative colitis, ankylosing spondylitis, lupus, rheumatoid arthritis, and psoriasis (Song). If you are experiencing chronic stress, your body is under relentless chemical assault.

But where the body produces "stress hormones" when a person feels under threat, it secretes equally powerful "relaxation hormones" when feeling good. These chemicals include serotonin, oxytocin, dopamine, and GABA chemicals. If you can calm down your nervous system enough to produce relaxation hormones, stress-induced physical symptoms will not only disappear; they will be replaced with a deep sense of well-being and a generally healthier body.

What does this have to do with your back pain and surgical choices? The bottom line is that a hyper-vigilant, fired-up nervous system increases your sensitivity to pain, and must be taken into account when deciding on treatment options—especially spine surgery, where there is no turning back.

The Treatment Grid

To summarize, the crucial factors when deciding whether to have spine surgery are the source of your pain and the status of your nervous system and body chemistry.

The source of your pain can be either structural or non-structural:

I. Structural:

–   Identified anatomical abnormality on an imaging study,

–   Symptoms that match the identified abnormality

II. Non-structural:

–   No identified anatomical abnormality,

–   Symptoms that don't match an identified abnormality

The status of your nervous system and body chemistry can be:

A. Calm nervous system

B. Stressed, hyper-vigilant, with sustained elevated levels of stress hormones

Depending on your individual situation, you'll fall into one of these four patient categories:

IA—Structural source of pain with a calm nervous system

IB—Structural source or pain with a stressed nervous system

IIA—Non-structural source of pain with a calm nervous system

IIB—Non-structural source of pain with a stressed nervous system

We have created a chart called a Treatment Grid, containing these four patient categories. If you understand your situation well enough to identify your place within the Treatment Grid, you will hold the key to the right decision about spine surgery. In the next chapter you will learn how to determine where you belong in the Grid.

	A CALM	B STRESSED
Type I STRUCTURAL	IA STRUCTURAL/ CALM • Surgery is an option • Simple prehab	IB STRUCTURAL/ STRESSED • Surgery is an option • Structured prehab
Type II NON- STRUCTURAL	IIA NON-STRUCTURAL/ CALM • Surgery not an option • Simple rehab	IIB NON-STRUCTURAL/ STRESSED • Surgery not an option • Structured rehab

The Treatment Grid

The Treatment Grid shows the categories in which surgery is a viable option, as well as other recommended treatments. Later in the book I will describe all these treatments options, including details of the most-performed surgeries.

CHAPTER 2

Getting on the Grid

YOUR FIRST STEP IN DECIDING whether to have spine surgery is to determine which quadrant of the Treatment Grid most closely resembles your condition. You will need to find out whether the source of your pain is structural (Type I) or non-structural (Type II), and whether your nervous system is calm (A) or stressed (B). (See the Treatment Grid on previous page.)

Structural or Non-structural?

Can surgery resolve the source of your pain? If an anatomical abnormality shows up on an imaging study (MRI, CT scan, or x-ray); and the accompanying symptoms exactly correspond to the abnormality; the answer is "yes." But hold on. Every anatomical abnormality has the potential for causing symptoms, but not all actually do. Also, even if a structural source *is* causing symptoms, they may be resolvable with non-surgical treatment.

For details about your diagnosis, read Chapter 3: The Source of Your Symptoms, and the relevant parts of Appendix A: Know Your Diagnosis. You will need this information to confirm whether the source of your pain is Type I (structural) or Type II (non-structural).

Type I's: Not so Fast.

If you determine that your source of pain is structural, you need to consider the following equally important factors.

1. Severity of the pain: Is the potential benefit worth the risk?

Pain is a mysterious thing. There is no way of accurately quantifying it, and pain thresholds differ widely, not only among people, but also from day to day within the same person. Everyone has good days and bad days. The important thing is to honestly assess the impact of your pain on your quality of life, and whether it is worth the risks of spine surgery. I have seen the simplest of cases go wrong with devastating consequences; and complex cases have even higher rates of serious complications. Since you are the one in pain, only you can decide whether it's worth a potentially life-changing complication. If your pain is mild and tolerable, I highly recommend first pursuing the non-surgical treatment options in presented in Chapter 7. There is nothing to lose and everything to gain.

2. Am I an A or a B?

Are they operating on your pain or your anxiety? Anxiety is the body's chemical response to a physical threat, real or imagined. The deeply unpleasant sensation gets your attention, with the intent to elicit evasive action so that you avoid the threat. Although surgically removing a structural source of pain may relieve some anxiety, it doesn't eliminate it. The key to reducing anxiety is training your body to secrete less stress hormones. There is so much data supporting the fact that anxiety compromises surgical outcomes, that several papers have pointed out that there is no need for further research on it (Edwards).

3. Do I have chronic pain?

When you perform procedures of any magnitude in the presence of untreated chronic pain, you will induce chronic pain at the new surgical site 20 – 60% of the time, with a 5 – 10% chance of the pain becoming permanent (Perkins). Chronic pain as a complication of surgery is rarely discussed, although it is a devastating complication.

4. The chances and consequences of failure

You need to understand the actual risks of any operation in general and yours in particular. In addition to the long list of complications that can occur during a procedure, there are possible long-term effects, such as having to return to the OR because of technical problems with the first operation. There is always a chance of your spine breaking down above or below a fusion. This can manifest as a fracture; a bend to the front or side; or a disc rupture that compresses the cord or nerves. Understanding the potential downside is critical in deciding whether the level of your pain is worth the risk. Chapter 8: Beware the IB Group: Failed Back Surgery, covers a few of the more common downsides of surgery, although this book can't possibly describe them all.

5. Is the magnitude of the operation appropriate?

There is a tendency for both surgeons and patients to opt for a larger, "definitive" operation rather than the simplest one that would get the job done. As a rule, the best choice is to perform the least invasive procedure possible. Failure of a major procedure, such as a multiple level fusion, results in greater negative consequences. Consult Appendix B: Know Your Procedure, to acquaint yourself with the scope and risks of the procedure recommended for your structural problem. Is a smaller procedure an option? If you have only moderate pain, a simple operation may be worth the risk of surgery; but a major one may not be.

Type II's: Hard Stop Here.

Surgery is off the table. If your health provider cannot clearly identify your source of pain on an imaging study, it is not amenable to surgery, period. You can't fix what you can't see. If your surgeon tells you that surgery is not indicated, let it go. It is fine to get another opinion or two, but don't go looking for a surgeon who will agree to perform surgery on you. You will find one.

For example, "degenerative disc disease" (not an actual disease but a normal, age-related deterioration of the tissue between vertebrae), is a common diagnosis that is used as a justification for surgery. However, it is not a reliable source of back pain (Boden) and does not respond to surgery (Carragee).

Patients who discover they are in the Type II group tend to get discouraged. Many believe that, not only will no one understand the depth of their suffering; but neither is there any hope for resolving it. It is actually great news to learn you have no apparent structural abnormalities that require surgery. It means you can take control of your recovery, using an assortment of low-risk treatments we like to call "non-operative, structured care." They work so well that many of my Type I patients, who came in with conditions I had routinely operated on in the past, canceled surgery because their pain disappeared during their self-directed, structured care program. These non-surgical treatments will be introduced in Chapter 7.

Calm or Stressed?

What is the status of your nervous system? This assessment is more personal than determining your source of pain. Even if you are typically someone who copes well with stress, carefully consider the impact of sustained anxiety, major losses, and prolonged pain.

If you are in a constant hyper-vigilant state, the sustained presence of stress chemicals can cause a myriad of physical symptoms, which are described in Chapter 6: Understanding Chronic Pain. You can regard these symptoms as indicators of the state of your nervous system. For example, you may not feel anxious or upset; but you may have ringing in your ears (tinnitus), stomach cramps (irritable bowel syndrome), migraine headaches, or any number of other ailments.

If your nervous system is "fired up," if you are struggling with difficult life situations in addition to your pain, if you are having a hard time coping with your pain, if you are anxious about your diagnosis, your future, etc.—then you are in the Type B group. You are at a greater risk for a less-than-optimal surgical result, no matter how appropriate or technically correct the procedure.

On the other hand, if you are relaxed and coping well with life's challenges, your chemical makeup is much different than that of the hyper-vigilant patient. Your body is functioning at a higher level and your chances of a successful surgical outcome are greater. If this sounds like you, you belong in the "A" column of the Treatment Grid.

Chapter 4, The State of Your Nervous System, will provide helpful insights for deciding whether you are an "A" or "B" on the Treatment Grid.

Type B's: Don't Mess with Stress.

Operations on patients with over-sensitized nervous systems are less successful and more risky. A poor surgical outcome can worsen your pain—perhaps permanently (Perkins). If you are a "B," calm down your nervous system (move to the "A" group) before considering surgery. The tools discussed in Chapter 7 will guide you towards the A group. If you are extremely anxious, you might be wise to seek help and support, whether or not your condition is amenable to surgery.

CHAPTER 3

The Source of Your Symptoms

SPINE SURGERY IS AN OPTION ONLY if your problem is structural and originates from the spine. There are treatment options for non-structural sources of pain, but they do not include spine surgery. Once you understand the principles that distinguish structural from non-structural sources of symptoms, you will be closer to making an informed decision about surgery and other treatment options.

Trying to Fix a Normal Spine

Robert was a 58-year-old successful businessman who had been experiencing severe low back pain (LBP) for five years. He had enthusiastically tried all kinds of therapies before succumbing to what had been suggested to him as a surgical solution. I saw him about a year after he had undergone a laminectomy, a procedure where a piece of a vertebra is removed in order to relieve compression of a nerve. He was now worse off than before. Not only did he suffer even more LBP, he now had unrelenting leg pain in the distribution of the nerve that had been decompressed. The really shocking thing, though, was when I examined his pre-operative MRI and I found no compression of the nerve prior to surgery. His spine had been completely normal, with not even a hint of a bulging disc. In fact, his spine had looked twenty years younger than his actual age—before surgery.

I worked with Robert for over a year, using the structured-care rehab concepts covered in Chapter 7. Part of his problem was his anger about agreeing to the surgery and his unwillingness to let it go. His persistent anger maintained an elevated level of stress chemicals, facilitating nerve conduction and increasing his pain, a phenomenon that has been demonstrated in animal research (Chen). It was a vicious cycle. Despite my best efforts I wasn't able to help him move on.

To review, here is what we have established about the two sources of pain in the human body:

Structural (Type I):

- An anatomic abnormality is visible on an imaging study;
- The symptoms (pain or neurological deficits, or both) correspond to the abnormality.

Non-structural (Type II):

- No anatomical abnormality is identified on an imaging test;
- The symptoms don't match the anatomic findings or are too vague to trace to a specific origin.

Appendix A provides details of the six most common spine diagnoses. Every specific spine diagnosis could be structural or non-structural. For example, a herniated disc as seen on an imaging study could have matching leg pain, which would define it as structural; or it could be asymptomatic, which would define it as non-structural.

The distinction between structural and non-structural problems rests on two factors: Anatomical findings and patterns of pain.

You might be wondering why we mentioned only pain and not neurological deficits such as weakness, numbness, and paralysis. The decision-making based on neurological symptoms depends on their severity and potential progression. It is usually not an elective situation, and therefore mostly outside the scope of this book. Neurological deficits will be discussed at the end of this chapter.

Anatomical Findings

When we examine an MRI, CT scan, or x-ray of your back, what exactly are we looking for? Basically, clear evidence of an anatomical abnormality—signs of injury or disease—particularly if it could be responsible for the pain pattern or neurological symptoms you are experiencing. Your symptoms must match the pathology to be considered a Type I scenario on the Treatment Grid.

Medicine has programmed most patients and health providers to believe that finding an anatomical source of pain is a victory. I believe the opposite is true. I hope you discover no structural problems. Your treatment options are more effective and less risky if you don't have to deal with a surgical procedure.

Structural Anatomy (Type I)

Anatomical characteristics that are likely to cause symptoms include:

- Instability: Abnormal or excessive motion (generally more than 3 or 4 millimeters in the lumbar spine and 2 to 3 mm in the neck) between vertebrae when you bend forward or backward.

- Compression:
  - A pinched nerve, with pain and/or neurological deficit in the pattern of that nerve (*radiculopathy*). The pressure can be from a bone spur or soft tissue within the spinal canal.

  - A compressed spinal cord that causes symptoms within the spinal cord (*myelopathy*). Cord symptoms are usually diffuse and more serious than pinched nerves. The spinal cord is more subject to injury and less likely to recover.

- A spinal deformity (curve) that is:
  - Decompensated (head not centered over the pelvis)
    - Forward (*kyphosis*)
    - Sideways (*scoliosis*)

- Both (*kyphoscoliosis*)
  - Collapsing (worse while upright compared to lying flat)
  - Progressive (more than 10 degrees)
- A spinal fracture that has not healed after four months, diagnosed by an MRI with a STIR (short inversion time recovery) sequence that reveals bleeding or hematomas. Factors that interfere with healing are:
  - Medications such as prednisone, anti-inflammatories, and others
  - Smoking
  - Obesity
  - Kidney failure
  - Severe osteoporosis

Non-structural Anatomy (Type II)

The following characteristics make an anatomic problem less likely to cause pain or neurological symptoms:

1. **Stability:** The segment of the spine is stable. The disc space may be completely collapsed, and the vertebrae essentially fused; but a disc that has minimal or no motion is not a source of pain, so surgery on that area would not be expected to alleviate any symptoms.

2. **Narrowing** around a nerve or the spinal cord *without* pain or neurological deficit in the pattern of that nerve or that level of the spinal cord. If there is fat or cerebrospinal fluid around the area in question, it is even less likely to cause symptoms.

3. **A spinal deformity that:**
   - Is balanced (your head is centered over your pelvis)
   - Remains stable between the lying down and upright positions
   - Has not changed for several years

4. **A spine fracture that has healed**, as indicated by repeat
    x-rays or an MRI with STIR images that show no fluid inside
    the vertebrae.

Incomprehensibly, and tragically, surgery is still being performed
on abnormalities with these non-structural characteristics, in the
face of strong evidence that they do not cause pain or neurological
deficits.

Patterns of Pain: Axial and Radicular

Axial Pain

Axial pain is pain located in the trunk of your body, from the base
of your neck to your pelvis, front back, or side. Pain centered in
your cervical (neck), thoracic, or lumbar spine is considered axial
pain. There are many causes of axial pain, but most are outside
the spinal column; therefore most axial pain is *not* treatable by
spine surgery. In terms of our Treatment Grid, most axial pain is
considered Type II (non-structural).

Structural Axial Pain (Type I)

In the presence of axial pain, a positive result on an imaging test
is more likely to reveal a very serious problem. Some diagnoses for
structural axial pain include:

- Instability
- Spinal deformity
- Malignant or benign tumors:
    - Primary (originating in the spinal cord) or
    - Metastatic (spread from other tissue)
- Infection of the vertebrae or disc space
- Traumatic acute fracture or an old fracture that hasn't
  healed
- Inflammatory or autoimmune diseases

Tumors and infections, although clearly different from each other,
have similar effects on the spine. Both are progressively destructive

processes that disrupt stability. The symptoms worsen over weeks to months until a critical amount of structural support is destroyed, at which time the spine becomes unstable. Usually, exiting nerves of the spinal cord are compressed, with resultant neurological deficits. If the problem is located in the cervical or thoracic spine, it can cause partial or complete paralysis. Both tumors and infections cause compression, but the infection additionally compromises the blood supply to the spinal cord by causing the small vessels to clot off. When complete paralysis occurs in this manner, it is permanent.

Acute traumatic fractures of the spinal column (those caused by a fall or other kind of force) are often structural, since they are clearly visible on an imaging test and the pain is usually centered over the injured area. The decision to perform surgery is left to the surgeon, based largely on whether the spine is stable. It is considered stable if there is minimal disruption of the bones and ligaments and little deformity or motion. It is considered unstable if there is gross movement or an associated neurological deficit. Excessive movement, termed translational instability, can be backwards or forwards. Vertebrae are usually parallel, but when one is tipped too far forward or backward with bending, it's called angular instability. The decision-making process around treatment for acute traumatic fractures is unique for every facture; it is complicated and requires a detailed conversation with the surgeon.

All the autoimmune disorders, such as rheumatoid arthritis, systemic lupus, and others, can cause damage to the spine from persistent inflammation. For example, rheumatoid arthritis can destroy the joint between the first and second cervical vertebra. The instability that results often requires a surgical fusion to decrease the pain and prevent neurological damage. During the inflammatory phase, while there is a lot of pain in the neck, it would be considered a non-structural problem without a surgical option. It becomes structural after the joint breaks down.

Another autoimmune disease is ankylosing spondylitis, which occurs most commonly in young males and presents with severe morning stiffness. All the soft tissues supporting the spine become inflamed, and eventually the entire spine spontaneously fuses into a solid piece of bone from neck to pelvis, earning the condition the nickname "bamboo spine." This is definitely a structural problem; however, surgery is indicated only if there is a fracture or significant deformity.

Ideally, autoimmune disorders will be discovered early, before they damage the spine. And there's no reason why they shouldn't be: Inflammation shows up in blood tests well before structural problems emerge.

An examination of diagnoses for structural axial pain is beyond the scope of this book. The condition is not very common; but for axial pain with structural origins, the surgical decision-making is mostly in the hands of your surgeon.

Red Flag Symptoms

There is one thing you can do, however: Be on the lookout for "red flag symptoms" associated with axial pain. If you have any of these, you must undergo the required diagnostic tests to rule out problems. Although this is the responsibility of your physician, these red flags could be missed in a busy clinic. Be sure to tell to your medical team if any items in the following list apply to you. If no one seems to be listening, be persistent.

- High energy injury (extreme force causing massive damage)
- History of infection
- Travel to a foreign country
- Fever, chills, night sweats
- Unexplained weight loss
- Generalized fatigue or weakness
- Acute onset of pain in a patient older than 50 or younger than 20
- History of osteoporosis
- Pain much worse at night
- History of cancer
- Low trauma spine fracture in a patient under 40 (Normally a lot of force is required to fracture a strong bone.)
- High-level performer forced to quit his or her passion

Fortunately, very little axial pain can be attributed to structural sources. We can determine the origin of lower back pain only 5 – 15% of the time (Nachemson).

Fracture Caused by a Low-Energy Accident

During my first year in practice I treated a 60-year-old farmer who had been rear-ended in a low-speed car accident. He came in with a compression fracture of his 8th thoracic vertebrae (T8), but the amount of trauma did not seem severe enough to cause a fracture, and his pain persisted longer than I thought it should. So I ordered an MRI scan of his thoracic spine, which revealed a tumor in the body of thoracic 8. A biopsy confirmed that it was malignant metastatic lung cancer. The patient's fracture was stable enough to be treated in a brace while he received radiation and chemotherapy for the tumor.

Often the first symptom of cancer is a spine fracture. The tumor invades and destroys the internal architecture of the vertebrae and weakens it to the point where it will either break spontaneously or fracture from minimal trauma. This is so common that I made it a practice of obtaining an MRI scan on almost every fracture I treated.

High School Football Star Forced to Give up Sports

I'll never forget the 17-year-old, 4-star high school athlete who had been experiencing pain in his tailbone for about six months. It was during the early years of my practice. He had seen four physicians, been to the ER several times, and was always sent home without much of a workup. Granted, tailbone pain is fairly common, and he didn't appear ill. But there were several red flags hinting of a serious problem. It hurt more at night, he had not experienced any trauma to the area, and the pain was severe enough to prevent him from being the starting quarterback for his football team.

I ordered an immediate CAT scan, which is highly sensitive of pelvic pathology. It revealed a tumor the size of softball at the tip of his sacrum. The cell type was that of a chordoma, a highly malignant cancer that can be cured only if caught early enough for it to be completely excised. Only a few centers in the country perform this extremely complex operation. Sadly, by the time I saw him, it was too late; he passed away six months later.

From this tragedy we can learn several lessons. The patient should always have a thorough history taken. In the student's case, had just one of his doctors acknowledged the warning signs, performed a simple rectal exam, and ordered diagnostic testing, the cancer could have been spotted before it was inoperable.

Non-structural Axial Pain (Type II)

Axial pain is usually widespread, vague and migratory. Since it is so diffuse, just by its nature it is almost impossible to attribute it to an anatomic source. Therefore, patients with this pattern of pain generally fall into the Type II group.

The most perverse violation of this principle is that of claiming degenerative disc disease is causing axial pain, when it has been shown repeatedly that disc degeneration does not. Degenerative disc disease is discussed in detail in Appendix A.

How can your imaging test reveal *no* abnormality to explain your symptoms, when you are in relentless pain? One reason is that your soft tissues are loaded with pain receptors—over a million per square inch. Anyone who has experienced tennis elbow, plantar fasciitis, rotator cuff tendonitis, or any other soft tissue inflammation knows how excruciating and prolonged the pain can be.

When chronic pain arises from soft tissues, no imaging test can pinpoint the source of pain. MRIs can sometimes reveal fluid that appears with acute tears and irritations. Palpating the area (examining with hands), observing when the pain increases and decreases depending on the patient's movements, and considering the circumstances around the onset of pain, we can form a fairly accurate diagnosis. A patient may have engaged in a new repetitive activity or decided to begin an aggressive exercise regimen. In that case, the diagnostic term would be "overuse syndrome." We still often order imaging tests to ensure a significant anatomical abnormality is not causing the symptoms.

Most of the pain complaints I have seen over my orthopedic career were traced to soft tissues. They included:

- Skin

- Fascia—the envelope of thin, leathery tissue that contains and defines muscle

- Tendons—rope-like tissue that attaches muscles to bone

- Ligaments—tissue that attaches bone to bone

- Joint capsules—pouches that contain synovial fluid, which lubricates each joint

- Intervertebral discs—one between each pair of adjacent vertebrae, providing a joint for movement, a ligament to hold them together, and a shock-absorbing effect

While soft tissue pain is not completely understood, we do know that the pain arising from these areas is often severe and prolonged. There are several reasons as why this is so:

- The soft tissues in the list above do not contain the rich blood supply found in muscles, skin, and internal organs. Therefore, the capacity for the body to heal when these soft tissues are inflamed is limited in comparison to our blood-rich organs.

- If there is inflammation, it takes weeks of a full therapeutic dose of anti-inflammatories to have an impact on the pain. Most people do not keep up with the dosing.

- After a prolonged bout of pain, the brain memorizes the neural circuit and can reproduce the pain sensations, often triggered by emotional stimuli, even after an initial injury has healed. At that point it doesn't matter how you treat the soft tissues (Hashmi).

- Most patients in pain stay active, which continues to irritate the painful tissues. Although it doesn't cause permanent damage, activity may prolong the healing process. One notable exception to this rule is gently engaging the painful areas of your body in light weight training with controlled repetitive movement, only not the activity that precipitated the pain. Using light weights and high repetitions, you can rapidly decrease pain and stiffness. I have prescribed this treatment for many patients with mid-thoracic pain, which tends to be persistent and annoying. It takes commitment, but most will experience relief over 3 – 6 months. I also advocate for all people to adopt an indefinite weight-training program for strength, flexibility and endurance.

Patients often worry that they might have a progressive structural problem if the pain grows worse. While it is important to rule out a structural problem, chances are it is chronic non-structural axial pain; it usually worsens gradually as the nervous system becomes sensitized (Gieseke). Tumors and infections progress rapidly over weeks to months. Having pain for years almost precludes these sources.

Radicular Pain

Radicular pain is pain that radiates into the arms or legs along the path of a spinal nerve root that is being compromised by pathology in the spinal column. Not all pain in the arms and legs originates from the spinal column, though. The term *radiculopathy* describes any condition following this pattern of pain.

Radicular symptoms appear from the shoulder down the arm, and from the buttocks down the leg. Since usually only one nerve is involved, symptoms are generally specific to that nerve and on one side of the body. This is in contrast to myelopathy (described later in this chapter), where the spinal cord is compromised, causing symptoms that are more widespread and vague.

There are four locations where spinal nerve root compression (stenosis) can occur and cause radicular symptoms. Their diagnoses are:

- Central stenosis—middle of the spinal (central) canal, resembling an hourglass
- Recess stenosis—immediately before the nerves leave the central canal
- Foraminal stenosis—the small openings in the side of the spine
- Extraforaminal stenosis—after nerves completely exit the spinal foramen

Central compression can cause myelopathy as well as radiculopathy in the cervical and thoracic spine. However, the other three areas of compression can cause only a radiculopathy. By the nature of the anatomy, radiculopathies almost always are in the cervical or lumbar spine. Thoracic problems are less common, as those problems usually occur within the central canal, causing a thoracic myelopathy. Possible radicular symptoms include:

- Localized numbness or tingling (although it's occasionally generalized)
- Pain in the distribution of the nerve(s). Usually the pain is on one side of the body.
- Isolated numbness and/or muscle weakness (occasionally on multiple levels)

Specifically, there are no myelopathic spinal cord symptoms or findings. Usually radicular pain travels along the path of the corresponding nerve and lasts either for minutes, hours, or constantly. If your leg or arm pain has any of the following characteristics, it is probably not a radiculopathy:

- The entire leg or arm hurts.
- The pain moves around, from day to day or within the same day.
- The symptoms are mostly numbness or tingling, not pain. The exception is when the symptoms are caused by pressure on the spinal cord (myelopathy).
- The pain is a quick, intermittent shooting pain, possibly severe.

Cervical Radiculopathy of the Left 6th Nerve

Many years ago, I was skiing in deep powder with a friend. He sat back on his skis, caught an edge and flipped over, landing on his head. Although the snow was deep and soft, his neck snapped back, and he experienced pain and numbness that traveled down the side of his arm and forearm into his thumb. This is the exact pathway of the 6th cervical nerve root. It resolved in about an hour; but whenever he is in a dental chair with his head back, his symptoms reoccur, until the staff provides a small pillow to keep his neck flexed. He never had an imaging study, but clinically he has either a bone spur or ruptured disc compromising the foramen (boney hollow between vertebrae through which spinal nerves run) between the 5th and 6th cervical vertebrae. Foramen narrow when the neck is tipped backwards.

In contrast to axial pain, the source of radicular and myelopathic symptoms are more likely to be structural—either from a pinched nerve or a compressed spinal cord. Frequently myelopathy and radiculopathy are accompanied by non-structural axial pain. However, if you undergo surgery for structural radiculopathy or myelopathy, it is *not* likely to relieve axial pain in your neck or back.

Compression of a peripheral nerve usually causes neurological deficits in a radicular pattern. This and other neurological deficits will be discussed at the end of this chapter.

Structural Radicular Pain (Type I)

First, in order for the radicular pain to be considered structural, it must manifest along the exact distribution of the nerve with the known spinal compression. For example, pain from the 5th lumbar (L5) or first sacral nerve (S1) must run along the sciatic nerve, down the side or back of the leg or calf, top or bottom of the foot, the big toe—or any combination of the above. Occasionally, the pain will be down both legs; but usually the symptoms are present in only part of the pathway. Many patients experience it only on the side of the calf or in the buttocks area. When I had my own bout with sciatica, my pain was only in my big toe.

If the third or fourth lumbar nerve (L3 or L4) is being pinched, the pain must travel along the femoral nerve path, down the front of the leg or in the groin. Both sciatic and femoral pain patterns are considered structural radicular.

Second, radiculopathy symptoms often are positional. If they get worse when you stand and walk, and disappear when you sit down, that means the canal or foramen is narrowing in the upright position and widening when you are sitting. Similarly, arm pain gets worse looking up and better looking down. Increased pain while sitting implies that there is soft disc rupture in the lower back. Sitting creates more pressure within the disc than when standing.

Third, true radicular pain is sustained, as opposed to sharp, shooting pain that comes and goes, no matter how frequently. If a nerve is compressed, the pressure doesn't let up; so the pain doesn't, either.

Radicular pain is often more severe than axial pain and will bias the decision toward surgery. Fortunately, these structural symptoms usually respond to surgical intervention. However, if there is severe axial pain accompanied by only mild radicular pain, there is a good chance the radicular pain is referred pain—pain that travels from the back or neck into the arm or leg through the soft tissues. If this is the case, not only will the axial pain remain after surgery, but also will the referred radicular pain.

Spinal cord tumors within the canal or within the cord are always a worry. These are tricky because they can cause almost any pain or neurological symptom, including radicular pain. I recall one case where a lumbar fusion was performed at the L5-S1 (the lowest level of the spine) for leg pain. The patient's symptoms were primarily radicular. It seemed like a reasonable choice except for a couple of suspicious observations: The constriction of the nerves wasn't severe enough to explain the leg pain, and the protein levels within the patient's cerebrospinal fluid (CSF) were over 100 (normal < 20). The patient had an undetected tumor in his spinal cord at the level of his 5th and 6th thoracic vertebra. The high CSF protein, in retrospect, was a major clue. The blood pressure changes during surgery compromised the blood supply around the tumor, causing infarction (tissue death) in the spinal cord. The patient woke up paraplegic. He should have had some signs of myelopathy, since the tumor was a thoracic lesion affecting his spinal cord. He did not.

Non-spinal Structural Sources that Create Radicular Pain Patterns

We have defined sources of structural pain as anatomy that can be identified on an imaging study, with symptoms that match the imaged anatomy. We have stated that pain sources must be structural in order to be considered for surgery. However, this is not to say that all structural causes of radicular pain are amenable to spine surgery. Some examples of non-spine structural problems causing a radicular pattern of pain are:

- Chondromalacia of the patella: A softening of the cartilage behind the knee, this condition can be responsible for pain under the kneecap. Occasionally, however, a similar pain pattern can arise from the 3rd lumbar nerve (L3), which travels directly to the knee. The diagnosis of chondromalacia of the patella is made by a careful history and a physical exam. There is no specific diagnostic imaging test to help identify this diagnosis.

- Hip arthritis: A common structural problem, but not a spine issue. It can cause severe pain down the front of the leg. I have seen several patients who underwent futile spine surgeries for this pain. Hips should be routinely included in all spine x-rays to rule out arthritis before undergoing spine surgery.

- Pelvic tumors: A tumor of the sciatic notch, for example, can cause radicular pain down the back of the leg; bladder cancer, down the front of the leg. Half of all metastatic (cancerous) spine tumors cause only radicular (leg or arm) pain.

- Pancoast tumors (lung cancer): This tumor at the apex of the lung can cause pain or neurological deficits down the arm.

Bladder Cancer

Henry was a construction laborer who had been suffering from a work-related injury for many years. He was disabled, and took high-dose narcotics. I saw him several times over the years and was sure there was nothing we could do surgically to improve his pain. He had also been bounced around the medical and Worker's Compensation systems.

About six months before one return visit to my office, he developed severe pain down the front of his leg and groin. These were new complaints. With his history of chronic pain, no one took him seriously and no work-up was done. Knowing his baseline symptoms and noticing the distinct change, I worked him up with a lumbar MRI, which showed no new findings. Henry was also experiencing a lot of pain at night, which is a worrisome symptom for cancer. Upon learning this I immediately followed up with a CT scan of his pelvis. It showed that his femoral nerve was encased in a large bladder cancer. Sadly, he passed away a few months later.

Non-structural Radicular pain (Type II)

Several patterns of pain can arise from soft tissues and from other diseases. Here are some examples of non-structural causes of radicular pain.

- Shingles, or herpes zoster, can cause severe pain down the path of any nerve. Usually, raised spots along the nerve path give away the diagnosis; but there may only one small lesion, or none at all.

- Brachial plexitis is a condition in which there is diffuse inflammation of the nerves exiting the spine in the neck. Although the inflammation can be seen on special MRI scans, its cause is unknown. The condition is usually manifested by severe, widespread pain in one arm and weakness in several muscles. The same problem in the lumbar spine is called lumbar plexitis and is much less common. This is a tough diagnosis to deal with but the good news is that it usually resolves on its own in 12 –18 months.

- Diabetic neuritis is poorly controlled diabetes that directly affects and inflames nerves. It may affect one or several nerves.

- Multiple sclerosis is a destructive autoimmune disease whose lesions can attack any part of the nervous system and create any symptom.

- Iliotibial (IT) band syndrome ("runners' knee") is an overuse injury of the connective tissues of the outer thigh and knee. (See the case study below.)

- A hyper-sensitized nervous system can cause one nerve to fire. Since the pain is so specific to the nerve, it clinically seems like there should be a structural problem causing it.

Referred pain can travel from the back or neck down the arm or leg via the webs of tiny nerves located in the fascial tissues surrounding muscles. The pain is usually more diffuse and less severe than axial pain.

If your spine pathology does not seem severe enough to cause your symptoms, a more thorough diagnostic analysis should be performed to search for other sources.

Iliotibial (IT) Band Syndrome

Soft tissue pain can be as severe a pain as any. Mark was a 50-year-old laborer who developed a low-grade pain down the side of his right leg. I thought perhaps it was an irritation of his 5th lumbar nerve root, which travels along that path. The pain pattern fit that of a structural radicular problem. When his pain suddenly spiked, we urgently admitted him to the hospital for pain control. He could barely stand up. We ordered another lumbar MRI, which I was positive would show a compressed fifth lumbar nerve; but the scan was normal. Upon re-examining him I discovered that applying pressure on the skin along the side of his leg caused severe pain.

He had an inflamed IT band, a fascial layer extending from the top of the pelvis down the side of the leg, attaching to the tibia (shin bone) just below the knee. Rich in pain fibers, fascia is the thin layer of tissue that encompasses and contains muscle. It also is the tissue that transitions from muscles to tendons, which attach muscle to bone.

The IT band contributes to stabilizing your hip and leg while walking, and it absorbs a lot of repetitive forces. A common source of leg pain particularly in runners and bicyclists, the band may become irritated along its whole length or only in spots. It is flat, but wide and long, so the pain can be intense. Think of all those millions of pain receptors per square inch.

With Mark we used a combination of pain control, ice, anti-inflammatories, and stretching to resolve his pain, but it took three days before he could leave the hospital. IT band pain is challenging to treat because the patient wants to keep moving. Usually it takes months to completely calm it down.

I have seen several cases where spine surgery was performed

to take pressure off the fifth lumbar nerve root when the actual diagnosis was iliotibial band syndrome. Of course the surgery wasn't helpful: The pre-operative imaging studies did not show any compression of the nerves.

One of my former fellows was told by a staff surgeon at a teaching hospital to sign a patient up for a spine fusion based only on the x-ray and MRI. The films revealed a small bony defect, but there was no nerve compression or instability. The surgeon had not seen or examined the patient, who was 35 years old. My fellow talked to the patient and did a thorough physical examination. It turned out he had bilateral iliotibial band tendonitis. Not only would he have not responded to surgery; but also the stress between the fusion and normal spine would be certain to break down during his lifetime, given his young age.

Neurological deficits

Neurological symptoms are almost always manifested in the extremities, and they include numbness, weakness, tingling, burning sensations, and bowel or bladder dysfunction—often occurring in different combinations.

There is always a reason for a neurological deficit. The cause can be structural—a lesion causing compression of the neural elements inside or outside the spinal canal. Or there may be a neurological condition directly affecting the nervous system. If the symptoms involve only peripheral nerves, it is considered a radiculopathy, described earlier in this chapter. Radiculopathy is one of three categories of symptom patterns that can result from compression of neurological tissues. The other two are myelopathy and cauda equina syndrome.

Myelopathy

Your spinal cord begins at the base of your skull and ends at the top of your lumbar spine at the level of the first lumbar vertebra (L1). Below L1, numerous nerve roots are floating in cerebrospinal fluid (CSF) down to your sacrum (center of the pelvic ring). Central compression of the spinal canal in the cervical and thoracic spine will create spinal cord symptoms called *myelopathy*.

Myelopathy is the set of symptoms originating from compromise to the spinal cord from many causes, including degenerative stenosis, ruptured discs, vascular injury, infection, and tumors within spinal cord tissue. Spinal cord tissue is similar to brain tissue and considered part of the central nervous system (in contrast to the peripheral nervous system). It's extremely sensitive to any insult and does not predictably recover. Therefore, when there are myelopathic symptoms, the surgical decision-making is much more aggressive; if you lose function, it may not return, or can take a very long time.

The symptoms of a myelopathy are different in the cervical, compared to the thoracic spine. The rib cage stabilizes most of the thoracic spine, so disc ruptures are rare at the upper thoracic levels. Problems in this area usually arise from major problems such as fractures, tumors or infections. Signs of a thoracic myelopathy include bilateral leg weakness, numbness or clumsiness. Bowel and bladder functions can range from lack of function to being spastic and overactive. There can be migratory (moving) or diffuse (widespread) pain. In fact, the symptoms can be so vague as to make thoracic spinal cord compression difficult to diagnose. Any time both legs exhibit unexplained neurological symptoms and the lumbar spine pathology is unremarkable, the thoracic spine should be examined.

Cervical myelopathy occurs more commonly than thoracic myelopathy because there is more motion in the neck. The signs and symptoms are easier to recognize. Slight burning in the fingertips of both hands, and/or a feeling of numbness in both palms can be early symptoms. The hands or arms may become weak. Problems with dexterity, such as writing, buttoning shirts, or tying shoes come later. More worrisome signs include unsteadiness, difficulty walking, irritable bladder, and falling. Isolated pain in the arms and legs is rare. Generally, the progressive neurological symptoms drive the surgical decisions.

Cauda Equina Syndrome

Below the tip of the spinal cord is the cauda equina (Latin for "horse's tail"). The sac of cerebrospinal fluid (dural sac) in the lumbar spine contains the nerves that make up the femoral nerve, sciatic nerve, and those that go to the bowel and bladder. These nerves take up less space in the central lumbar canal than does the spinal cord in the cervical and thoracic spine. Therefore only a large lesion will cause enough compression to cause neurological compromise. Although rare, a large massive disc rupture may cause a rapid onset of bowel and bladder dysfunction called cauda equina syndrome. There is usually accompanying leg numbness and weakness. This is a true surgical emergency.

The more common cause of bladder urgency and frequency is interstitial nephritis, also called spastic bladder, or irritable bladder syndrome, and has nothing to do with structural sources. It is a common symptom of many caused by a sensitized nervous system, discussed in Chapter 4. It is up to your doctor to figure this out. With this condition, there is no numbness or tingling in the groin area, no leg weakness, bowel function is unchanged, and usually the compression of the nerves is not impressive. The symptoms resolve with an effective rehab program that desensitizes the patient's nervous system.

Not Cauda Equina Syndrome

Several years ago, I was asked by one of my partners to perform an urgent lumbar surgery on an older woman because he felt that she had a cauda equina syndrome. Her MRI scan did show significant compression of the nerves at the level of the 3rd and 4th lumbar vertebra. However, these were old findings with nothing to indicate anything had changed. I also didn't feel the constriction was severe enough to cause neurological deficits and she had no numbness in the groin area or weakness in her legs.

When I spoke to her, she related that she was under extreme personal stress and had been recently diagnosed with an autoimmune disorder. I elected not to perform surgery in spite of pressure from my partner and her friends. She engaged in the structured rehab program and three months later her bladder symptoms resolved. A year later she was thriving.

The reason I am addressing neurological issues is that I have seen spine surgery performed on pathology that wasn't severe enough to cause the neurological symptoms. The correct diagnosis was delayed. For example, a neck fusion was performed in an older woman for progressive weakness. There was some narrowing, but it turned out that she had Amyotrophic Lateral Sclerosis (ALS), commonly known as Lou Gehrig's disease. The disease affects the motor neurons in the spinal cord, and patients usually succumb when the rib cage muscles become too weak to support breathing. She passed away a couple of months later.

Another disease that primarily affects the muscles, causing diffuse weakness and pain, is polymyalgia rheumatica, which inflames muscle fibers. The tragedy of missing this diagnosis is that it is easily treated with steroids. The only test needed to diagnosis it is a blood test that measures inflammation.

Every neurological deficit should be carefully attended to. Failing to perform a thorough workup on someone with neurological symptoms is dangerous. One mentally compromised 30-year-old gentleman presented to the emergency room three times after a fall because he was experiencing balance problems. He was sent home each time because he was "acting unusual." The ER staff, feeling that the patient was exaggerating his complaints, did not perform a thorough neurological examination. Three days later he became quadriplegic. He had been living with bone spurs in his neck that were pressing on his spinal cord. The fall had jammed them into his cord, and delayed swelling caused severe damage.

ALS, not Spinal Stenosis

Ron was a 46-year-old, physically fit mason who was referred to me for surgery for spinal stenosis (narrowing of the spinal canal) between his 3rd and 4th lumbar vertebrae (L3-4). He had no pain; only increasing weakness in both legs, in nerves originating from several levels of his spine. However, his MRI scan showed only moderate stenosis, and there was still cerebrospinal fluid around the nerves. It was clear that there was not enough constriction of the nerve to cause any weakness, and certainly not at all the levels he was experiencing.

I referred Ron to a neurologist who quickly made the diagnosis of Amyotrophic Lateral Sclerosis (ALS). This is a rapidly progressive neurological disease that directly affects the cell bodies of motor neurons in the spinal cord. Patients die from inability to breathe from weakened chest wall muscles and diaphragm. I had come close to performing a one-level laminectomy, but the clinical picture just wasn't right. I am grateful I hesitated. Ron certainly didn't need to compound his misery with unnecessary spine surgery.

Summary

The goal of this chapter is to provide an overview of types of sources of spinal pain to determine if you fit into the Type I (structural) part of the Treatment Grid or have a non-structural (Type II) source of your pain. Both the anatomic lesion and pain pattern define whether there is a structural problem or not.

The pattern of pain must match the anatomy in order for the source of the pain to be considered structural. Axial pain is rarely structural unless there is a significant anatomical abnormality and the pain is centered on that area. Radicular pain has a much higher chance of being from a structural spine source.

Medical decisions based on neurological deficits are more clear-cut: There is either a structural explanation or not. If there is an anatomical problem, the decisions are based on the degree as well as the progression of deficits. If neurological symptoms arise from a disease that affects the nervous system, surgery is not a choice.

CHAPTER 4

The State of Your Nervous System

A PERSON'S STRESS LEVEL HAS a marked effect on both your central and peripheral nervous systems. The central nervous system (CNS) consists of your brain and spinal cord. The peripheral nervous system (PNS) includes all other nervous system tissue—the nerves exiting your spinal cord, all sensory receptors, and sensory and motor neurons.

The secretion of survival "flight or fight" hormones such as adrenaline, cortisol and histamines affects every cell in the body, with the potential of creating over thirty physical symptoms. One of them, as demonstrated in laboratory animal studies, is increased speed of nerve conduction, which intensifies the sensation of pain (Chen). From a strict survival perspective, it makes sense: When the situation calls for it, you should be on high alert, in order to defend yourself and whoever else you're responsible for protecting. But the relentless bombardment of stress hormones takes a toll on your body.

Consider driving your car down the freeway at 70 mph in second or third gear, instead of cruising in fourth or fifth. How long do you think your over-extended engine would hold up? The same is true for your body. Not only will you suffer a multitude of physical symptoms manifested by the burden placed on your body; you will be operating with a weakened immune system. For example, a large study found a clear connection between chronic stress and autoimmune disorders such as rheumatoid arthritis, Crohn's disease, ulcerative colitis, ankylosing spondylitis, and psoriasis, among others (Song). Research results going back fifty years identify chronic stress as a risk factor for frequent and serious illnesses (Rahe), and a shortened life span (Torrance).

Am I in Category A (Calm) or B (Stressed)?

In this chapter you will increase your awareness of your stress levels and other factors that affect not only your physical discomfort, but also the outcome of your surgery, should you decide to have it. Only you can accurately assess the sensitivity of your nervous system. Is it calm enough to provide optimal conditions for solving your physical problems (Type A)? Or is it sensitized (Type B), which may hinder the outcome of your treatment?

If you are in the Type B group, your first order of business should be to work towards changing your body's chemistry—reducing stress hormone levels—and move into the Type A quadrant. But how? Outside help, in the form of a counselor or other supportive professional or program, is always a viable option; but you have many other choices. I've identified several effective stress-reduction activities you can initiate on your own, which you will learn about in Chapter 7, where we discuss the Direct your Own Care (DOC) program. These are safe, simple activities that have caused patients to cancel their surgeries and go pain-free, without risking further damage and more pain.

But first, you need to determine your place within the grid—whether you are a Type A or Type B.

Factors that Determine the State of Your Nervous System

1. **Quality of sleep.** Are you getting enough? Lack of sleep compromises every aspect of your treatment, whether it is surgical or non-operative care.
2. **Level of chronic stress.** Are you chronically anxious, frustrated, depressed, angry, fearful?

3. **Level of situational stress.** Are you dealing with an unusually difficult situation in your life, in addition to the problems created by your pain?

4. **Physical manifestations.** Are you experiencing random symptoms such as rashes, headaches, or tinnitus?

5. **Commitment to recovery.** Are you open-minded regarding learning about the nature of chronic pain and the principles behind solving it? Are you willing to commit to a long-term program that will resolve your pain and improve the quality of your life? Are you addicted to your pain or using it to your advantage? Believe it or not, people often become addicted to being in pain. One's medical condition can be powerful weapon, and the unwillingness to let it go is the one greatest obstacle to healing.

Considering these five areas is meant to give you a feel for the state of your nervous system and the extent to which protective (harmful when sustained) stress hormones are coursing through your body. This is crucial information for you to know. A hyper-vigilant nervous system negatively affects not only your pain and your surgical outcomes, but your overall quality of life as well.

Quality of Sleep

You might wonder what your sleep habits have to do with this conversation; but your quality of sleep probably has a greater impact on your nervous system than any other factor. It is also likely the easiest issue to correct. I feel so strongly about the role of sleep in predicting treatment outcomes that I insisted my patients maintained regular, restful sleep for at least six weeks before assessing their level of pain or deciding whether they needed surgery.

Sleep deprivation alters both your perception of pain and your capacity to cope with it. Neither can you heal properly without adequate sleep, as I have observed over several decades of treating thousands of patients.

By merely improving your quality of sleep, you might experience a dramatic decrease in your pain levels. I've seen 20 – 30% declines in many patients, and occasionally nearly complete cessation of pain. I remember one gentleman who had seen multiple physicians for over two years for chronic neck pain. He also had severe sleep issues, which his other physicians had not addressed. I started him on medications for sleep, and when he returned for his six-week appointment, his pain had completely resolved.

I had always assumed that it was a one-way relationship—that chronic pain inhibited restful sleep—and research supported this notion (Karaman). But a large 2014 study (Agmon) found that the reverse was also true: Lack of sleep induced chronic pain. While the relationship between sleep and chronic pain appears to be viciously cyclical, we are confident of one thing: Poor sleep escalates the misery of chronic pain. Even if you feel calm and you have no major stresses in your life, the combination of insomnia and chronic pain would place you on the Type B side of the grid.

Levels of Chronic Anxiety, Frustration and Depression

Everyone has stress in some form or another. But whatever your life situation or your environment, simply coping with day-to-day challenges such as meeting your basic needs and dealing with other people creates some degree of stress. Yes, you may be successfully surviving and maneuvering through today's complicated world; but the real question is, "What is your quality of life and sense of well-being?"

Regardless of your ability to prevail over life's challenges, you may not be aware of chronic anxiety, depression, frustration, or anger. All these emotions represent your reaction to stress, and you have a charged up nervous system, placing you in a Type B quadrant of the Grid. Using a reliable questionnaire can identify what's really going on and the impact of stress on your mood. If you're like most people, you are so used to being under stress that it has become your "normal" state, and you are too busy to notice. But while some stress is normal and even advantageous, chronic stress is not. Especially if you have chronic pain, use this simple mood questionnaire to help you reflect on what you might be feeling over the last few weeks.

Mood Questionnaire

These questions are about how you feel and how things have been with you *during the past four weeks*. For each question, please give one answer that comes closest to the way you have been feeling.

Circle the appropriate number to indicate the extent of the problem you are having with each of the following:

	None										Severe
Anxiety	0	1	2	3	4	5	6	7	8	9	10
Depression	0	1	2	3	4	5	6	7	8	9	10
Irritability	0	1	2	3	4	5	6	7	8	9	10

These 1 – 10 scales are not a validated research questionnaire. I used it for over 30 years on every new patient and my impression was that if someone rated themselves as a six or higher on at least one of the categories on the Mood Questionnaire, it indicated to me that I needed to find out more about him or her. There were often significant issues creating more than minimal stress, anxiety, frustration or anger (Type B, Hyper-Vigilant).

If you rated yourself 0, 1, or 2 on the mood questionnaire and have been suffering from prolonged chronic pain, I consider it a red flag. Can your mood really be that great after suffering for so long, failing again and again to resolve your pain, with no end in sight? You may be suppressing your thoughts and feelings, which only adds fuel to your already fired-up nervous system.

Remember that *everyone has some level of stress* just living a normal life, even without pain. When a body's stress level is such that it floods the nervous system with stress hormones, it produces a feeling of anxiety, the extreme being a panic attack. Even if you are in denial about your anxiety, your body will manufacture physical symptoms.

"I Am Not Stressed"

Georgia, a 64-year-old woman who had suffered from back pain for over fifteen years, had undergone four spine surgeries encompassing over half her spine before she became my patient. Her pain now radiated throughout her entire body, limiting her activities such that she could barely take care of her basic needs. On her intake questionnaire, she had rated her anxiety, depression and irritability levels as "zero"; and when questioned, stubbornly stuck to her story, "I'm fine. I don't have any stress." When I suggested that experiencing diffuse pain might be a significant source of stress, she became indignant and began yelling at me. When I suggested that just suffering from chronic pain was a major source of stress, she become even more upset. At the top of her lungs, she insisted that she was calm. She flatly refused when I requested that she merely learn about the neurological nature of chronic pain, the first step in the DOC program. I continued to work with her for a couple of years, never sure why she kept returning; but she never tried any of the non-surgical strategies that were so effective with other patients with severe chronic pain. Sadly, she never improved.

Often the person in the worst shape is the last to realize it. I'm hard-pressed to recall any patients who, after rating themselves as "zeros" on the stress scale, engaged in the non-surgical healing strategies available to them. Assess yourself with the knowledge that your mood affects all treatment outcomes (Linton).

Level of Situational Stress

Until a few years ago, I attributed my patients' symptoms to either (1) an anatomical problem that I might be able to solve with surgery; or (2) inflammation of soft tissues—muscles, tendons, fascia or ligaments. The conversation always centered on the physical aspect of the pain.

Then I happened to encounter four patients inside of two weeks with whom I had weirdly identical conversations. All men between the ages of 45 and 65, each had leg pain originating from an identifiable anatomical source in his spine, severe enough to warrant surgery. Each also circled at least an "8" on the anxiety scale and reported difficulty sleeping. When I inquired about their anxiety, one answered that his teenage daughter was seriously ill; another complained of weighty marital problems; the last two described difficult work situations, one with a boss who bullied him. All four of these patients had another common issue. They were all high-level professionals whose self-image didn't allow them to admit to themselves or others how much they were suffering.

I told each of them that, although I would love to immediately rid them of their leg pain with surgery, my bigger concern was their high level of anxiety and possibly the chronic nature of their pain. Recalling what went through my head during my own fifteen-year battle with pain and anxiety, I asked each of these patients if they could get rid of their pain or decrease their anxiety, what would they choose? Each of them grabbed his leg and asked, "Won't relieving the let pain decrease my anxiety?" I told them, "No." In fact anxiety usually worsens over time, regardless of the outcome of the surgery. All of them felt they could deal with the leg pain more easily than living with relentless anxiety. I explained that, although it may decrease for a few weeks after the surgery, there were too many other factors contributing to chronic anxiety that needed to be addressed before they saw a significant drop in their anxiety levels.

This set of encounters precipitated a huge shift in my thinking. As much as I knew how much pain and anxiety were linked, I had never realized that for many patients the pain relief they were seeking was for peace of mind.

When they realized how disruptive their anxiety was to their quality of life, all four of these men were willing to give the DOC program a try. Within weeks, as their anxiety levels dropped, their pain either disappeared or subsided enough to a level where they no longer considered surgery was necessary.

There are many effective treatments for anxiety, but surgery isn't one of them. If you are anxious, depressed, and angry now, think how you'll feel if you go through a surgery that fails to bring you relief of either your pain or anxiety. You will have lost another battle and another level of hope.

I have always been uncomfortable recommending surgery for a patient who was facing extreme personal adversity, and my encounters with those four gentlemen clarified why. After those two weeks, I began asking every one of my patients to answer the simple question, "Have you been under an unusual amount of stress over the last year?" The answer I typically received was a resounding "Yes," and often along with it, a harrowing story. I was amazed at the level of suffering people endured and how consistently physical pain accompanied their life crises.

Any painful situation where you feel trapped will fire up your nervous system, as your body automatically prepares to escape. Some of the more common causes of situational stress are:

- **Navigating through Workers' Compensation**—Those in state disability programs know how it feels to be at the mercy of a bureaucratic government system that can't respond to your needs and is constantly challenging the validity of your pain. Every aspect of your care is challenged, and employers are often unsympathetic Regardless of the legitimacy of your anger, however, it still adversely affects your pain, body, and general health.

- **Social isolation**—A large 2018 survey conducted on 20,000 people by Cigna, a prominent insurance company documented that 50 – 55% of the US population is socially isolated (Cigna). There are devastating mental and physical effects of loneliness (Hawkley). Social isolation stimulates an area of the brain close to that of chronic pain and causes the same chemical reaction as a physical threat (Eisenberger). Many of my patients have felt that re-engaging with family and friends is an important aspect of their journey out of pain.

- **Physical, emotional or sexual abuse**—Only 30% of Americans are raised in households that are relatively stress free. Over 35% are members of households that by any standards are chaotic and sometimes dangerous (Anda). Multiple studies document the finding that trauma experienced in childhood results in chronic diseases, including pain in adulthood (Dube).

- **Loss of a family member**—Especially traumatic when unexpected, such as accidental death or suicide.

"My Son Just Died."

George was a pleasant 78-year-old businessman who acted and looked half his age. He clearly described a specific pain down the side of one leg, how it became more severe when standing and walking, and disappeared when he sat. His MRI revealed a bone spur pushing on his fifth lumbar nerve root—an anatomical problem that perfectly matched his symptoms; so, it seemed like an easy fix to perform a one-level fusion. With his positive attitude and level of physical fitness, he was the ideal candidate for a procedure. I am not in the habit of making surgical decisions on the first visit; but there was nothing on his intake questionnaire that looked worrisome, and he was eager to resolve his condition, so it seemed safe to move ahead. In my estimation he was a classic Type IA: Calm, with a structural source of his symptoms.

As I began to leave the room to grab some paperwork, he murmured something about his son, who was his partner in the family business, having died of a heart attack a few months prior. I immediately put on the brakes.

"George," I said; "I'm not comfortable with you making a major decision in light of the situation. Why don't we wait a couple of weeks?" He agreed, and left with a copy of my book, *Back in Control,* which contains information on dealing with stress, chronic pain, post-operative pain and rehab. A week later he called and told me he wasn't interested in using the tools in the book; he just wanted to proceed with surgery. I asked him just to glance through the book and begin to engage in the expressive writing exercises before his next appointment. Again, he agreed, and in the meantime, I put him on the schedule for surgery.

When George appeared for his next visit, our final pre-operative consultation, we had a long conversation about the effects a major loss can have on a person's body. He asked if it was OK to postpone his surgery for a while.

One month later I saw him in my office, pain-free and fully functioning, having just re-activated his gym membership. He had continued to read the book but had not begun to use any of the suggested exercises. Now, I am well aware that reading my book or any book is usually not going to relieve pain. But for George, I believe that slowing down, talking to friends, and realizing the gravity of his loss were calming him down, and all were instrumental in resolving his physical pain. He was now focusing more on helping his wife with her grief.

Surgery may or may not relieve your arm or leg pain. It rarely solves neck or back pain. It certainly won't cure anxiety. But if you are in the grips of a major loss, you are (at least temporarily) a Type B and at a great risk to undermine the success of any surgery. Even if you are the kind of person, like George, who can still function while enduring unspeakable emotional pain, be careful. Give yourself a break and take some time before making the huge decision to have surgery.

Physical Manifestations of Stress

When your body is constantly bombarded with stress hormones, you develop physical symptoms. While these manifestations may be uncomfortable or downright torturous, they are helpful clues to the state of your nervous system. You can and should use your body's physical signals as a "body barometer"—an indicator of your levels of stress hormones.

My 15-year ordeal with chronic pain began quietly, going from the absence of any anxiety to a series of panic attacks, all within one day. Once the lid blew off, I could not put it back on and I began experience unrelenting progressive anxiety. It made no sense to me. Although my stress levels were high, they were no worse than "normal." I now know that emotional pain and physical pain are processed in the brain in a similar manner. If you don't feel the mental pain, your body will manifest physical symptoms. I had been experiencing migraine headaches, obsessive thought patterns, insomnia, burning sensations in my feet, tinnitus, and PTSD for many years. As an adult, my coping skill was "being tough" with a "bring it on" approach. I was a master at suppressing almost anything known for being cool under pressure. One not-so-complimentary nickname I earned was "The Brick."

I pushed myself relentlessly—some might say obsessively—to accomplish my many goals. But was I really "successful?" Eventually the same energy that pushed me up the hill tossed me down the other side. I lost almost everything, including my marriage and my job. Miraculously, I stumbled on a solution that relieved all my symptoms and sustains me to this day—as long as I continue to use the tools, I will describe in Chapter 7.

Even now, I suppress anxiety and frustration more than I would like to admit. And if I interrupt my practice of the strategies that I teach to my patients, within a week or so I begin to experience the physical symptoms that plagued me during my breakdown. For example, if I stop doing my expressive writing or working out at the gym, I may "feel" fine, but I become more reactive and my sleep quality drops. Small skin rashes appear on the backs of my wrists, my feet burn, and tinnitus returns. I now accept the fact that my body is chronically full of stress chemicals, even if my external circumstances are on an even keel. Even so, I make it a point to look for situations that may have triggered me; and when I re-engage in the healing practices, my symptoms abate quickly.

Sustained elevated levels of stress chemicals can result in a variety of symptoms, which can be grouped into four categories (Abbass, 2008):

- Striated-muscle tension—tension headaches, fibromyalgia (chronic, widespread pain and oversensitivity to pressure), backache, fatigue, shortness of breath

- Smooth-muscle tension—Irritable bowel syndrome, abdominal pain, nausea, migraines, bladder spasm

- Cognitive-perceptual disruption—visual blurring, mental confusion, memory loss, dizziness, pseudo seizures

- Conversion—falling, aphonia (loss of voice), paralysis, weakness

Dr. Howard Schubiner, a pain specialist and expert in the interdependence of environment and health, lists 33 symptoms that can arise from the body's chemical reaction to stress (Schubiner).

1. Heartburn, acid reflux GERD)
2. Abdominal pains
3. Irritable bowel syndrome (IBS)
4. Tension Headaches

5. Migraine Headaches

6. Unexplained rashes

7. Anxiety and/ or panic attacks

8. Depression

9. Obsessive-compulsive thought patterns

10. Eating Disorders

11. Insomnia or trouble sleeping

12. Fibromyalgia (FMA)

13. Back pain

14. Neck pain

15. Shoulder pain

16. Repetitive stress injury

17. Carpal tunnel syndrome (CTS)

18. Reflex sympathetic dystrophy (RSD)

19. Temporomandibular joint syndrome (TMJ)

20. Chronic tendonitis

21. Facial pain

22. Numbness, tingling sensations

23. Fatigue or chronic fatigue syndrome (CFS)

24. Palpitations

25. Chest Pain

26. Hyperventilation

27. Interstitial cystitis/ spastic bladder (irritable bladder syndrome)

28. Pelvic pain

29. Muscle tenderness

30. Postural orthostatic tachycardia (POTS)

31. Tinnitus

32. Dizziness

33. PTSD (Post-traumatic Stress Disorder)

24 Physical Symptoms

Susan, a psychiatrist in her 60's, contacted me about attending one of my workshops. On the intake questionnaire, which included Dr. Schubiner's list of 33 symptoms, she had checked off 24 of them. Her symptoms included tailbone pain after sitting more than 10-15 minutes, which had persisted over a span of ten years and prevented her from doing her job.

She had read my book and begun to use the expressive writing strategy for a few weeks. Although she had already experienced a slight shift in her mood, I wasn't optimistic because of the number of symptoms and how long she had been suffering. I didn't encourage her to make the trip to the workshop.

She attended the workshop anyway and immersed herself in the DOC process. We had a great time getting to know and work with each other. She kept diving in deeper into the DOC process, which taking charge of her care and personal life, exercising, forgiveness, awareness, and moving forward with her pain. She went back to work and over the next year her pain dramatically diminished. We stay in touch and although she has weathered some flare-ups, she is working part time, remarried, and living a full life. She was in terrible pain with all 24 of her symptoms being disruptive to her capacity to enjoy life. In retrospect, the key to her improvement was her willingness to learn engage in her own healing journey.

Use your physical symptoms as indicators that you are being triggered, and your nervous system is fired up—even if you don't feel stressed. I think everyone has at least three or four of these symptoms just from dealing with life.

Commitment to Recovery

On the surface, you might think it's ridiculous to ask yourself how committed you are to recovering. Who wouldn't want to get rid of pain? The medical director of my hospital's pain center taught me that the only thing holding people back from healing was their unwillingness to engage in the treatment process. Eventually, after experiencing countless patients who inexplicably refused to participate in their own healing, I concluded that many people simply do not want to give up their pain. I would spend hours trying to convince them to engage in proven treatment programs; but the harder I tried, the more emotional and combative our interaction would become. It is this whole dynamic—the unwillingness to let go and move forward—that is the greatest obstacle to healing.

Several reasons may explain why people may not want to heal. If you step back and think for a minute, you'll realize that pain is powerful. You are truly a victim. Others demand less of you and you expect less of yourself. You can hide behind it or you may demand others close to you take care of you. The impact of pain on the family is usually devastating. So, you feel powerful (it may or may not be real) and you don't want to give up. At the same time, you feel powerless from being in pain. It is a quandary.

Second, dealing with pain can become a way of life, a person's identity, even an "occupation." It may come with a high level of anxiety, but at least it's familiar, and that's a source of comfort. Change is likely to be met with resistance because it may produce even more anxiety. As a doctor who has walked in his patients' shoes, it did not surprise me that the harder I tried to convince people to take responsibility for their pain and care, the more resistant they became.

Thirdly, functional MRI research has revealed that the brains of people with chronic pain physically shrink (Seminowicz), resulting in decreased cognitive function. (IOM) It becomes difficult to think clearly and make good decisions. Fortunately, when the pain is resolved, the brain can quickly re-expand, returning the patient's capacity to engage in creative thinking.

A fourth possible reason some patients resist taking steps to cure their pain is that their thinking may be tainted by anger. Everyone feels angry at times, but chronic pain intensifies the emotion. When you are trapped by any circumstance, anger is always the next reaction to try to escape. Being engulfed in pain is especially unpleasant and Dr. Sarno referred to it as "rage" (Sarno). While their resistance might seem like mere stubbornness, angry patients may be understandably lashing out against their doctors, but it is also ultimately directed against themselves. Anger encompasses everyone in the vicinity.

Finally, anger contributes to obsessive, repetitive thought patterns, which can contribute to a patient's unreceptiveness to treatment. I call it "phantom brain pain." It is similar to phantom limb pain, where an arm or leg continues to hurt even after it has been amputated. Similarly, repetitive thoughts continue to cycle through the patient's consciousness long after they are helpful or even relevant. Uncontrollable thought patterns are not subject to rational interventions; but they can be weakened if the patient is the slightest bit open to the approaches we explore in Chapter 7.

In my experience, the person steeped in rage was rarely willing to engage in any purposeful healing process. Breaking through anger was the greatest challenge I faced in helping patients solve their pain problems.

I suppose the question "Am I willing to heal?" should be rephrased as "Am I willing to participate in my healing?" Patients who believe that a surgical procedure will solve all their problems—including the emotional ones—fall into the Type B classification. But if you have read up to this point, you are likely to participate in your recovery.

Not Sleeping and Not Willing to Learn

A forty-year-old patient, about 250 pounds of pure muscle, came to me for a surgical opinion about his low back pain. He had some mild disc degeneration, normal for his age, but not a cause of back pain; it had been recommended that he undergo a two-level fusion of the L4-5 and L5-S1 discs. During our conversation he revealed that he'd been sleeping only three to four hours a night for almost nine months. None of his medical team had addressed his insomnia. I explained to him that his sleep deprivation was severe, that it was unwise to make a decision regarding surgery in his condition and that he needed to first be treated for his sleep issues as part of a structured rehab program before proceeding with any further treatment. He said that, while he didn't want surgery, neither did he want to engage in any part of the structured program. No matter what I said, he refused. To me, a patient with such an attitude is untreatable. It took me years to realize that I was talking to irrational spinning neurological circuits and the conversations were always circular. This interaction is common and occurred daily in my practice. I learned to let go quickly. If I tried to reason with a patient in this state of mind, he or she would always become more upset. He never returned and I don't know the final outcome.

Summary

Now that you are aware of the factors that affect the state of your nervous system, you can determine whether you are Type A (handling stress and calm) or B (overwhelmed and hyper-vigilant).

You don't necessarily need to alleviate all your Type B characteristics before proceeding with an operation; but you should definitely try to find a way to gravitate towards Type A before having surgery, in order to optimize your results. There are many effective ways to calm down your nervous system, as you will read in Chapter 7.

SECTION 2: TAKE CONTROL

CHAPTER 5

Your Treatment Options

THE TREATMENT GRID PRESENTS the treatment options available to you, based on the source of your symptoms and the state of your nervous system. At this point you should have a fairly good idea of which quadrant of the Treatment Grid you fit into. This chapter will bring into focus the treatment paths available to you.

	A CALM	B STRESSED
Type I STRUCTURAL	IA STRUCTURAL/ CALM • Surgery is an option • Simple prehab	IB STRUCTURAL/ STRESSED • Surgery is an option • Structured prehab
Type II NON- STRUCTURAL	IIA NON-STRUCTURAL/ CALM • Surgery not an option • Simple rehab	IIB NON-STRUCTURAL/ STRESSED • Surgery not an option • Structured rehab

The Treatment Grid

Type IA—Structural Source/Calm Nervous System

Placement in the Type IA quadrant requires three criteria: 1) You have a structural abnormality identified by an imaging study; 2) that abnormality is the probable cause of your symptoms; and 3) you are coping reasonably well with your pain as well as your everyday challenges.

If you are a Type IA, you may be continuing work and remaining active; but pain is compromising your quality of life. If the pain is severe enough to warrant surgery, the outcomes are usually predictable, with satisfying pain relief. Once you have read about the relevant procedures in Appendix B, use the following questions to focus your decision:

- Is my pain severe enough to undergo any spine surgery?

- Do I fully understand the magnitude and negative aspects of the proposed procedure? Is it the least invasive option?

- Have I fully engaged in a structured treatment program to optimize my outcome or possibly avoid surgery?

Expect post-operative rehab to involve learning excellent posture and body mechanics, practicing exercises daily, and maintaining a long-term body-conditioning regimen to build up your strength. A combination of aerobic activity and weight training is usually recommended. Your spine will never be as strong as it was prior to surgery, but this rehab regimen will compensate for it.

Type IA patients typically are successfully treated with minimal use of medical resources, which may or may not include surgery. More information about their treatment paths can be found in my book, *Back in Control: A Surgeon's Roadmap Out of Chronic Pain* (Hanscom, 2016).

Ruptured Lumbar Disc

Jane, a 30-year-old construction worker, was injured on the job when she ruptured her disc between her fourth and fifth vertebrae (L4-5). It pinched the fifth lumbar nerve root, which travels down the side of the leg. Jane had endured leg pain for three months before undergoing a microdiscectomy, which took the pressure off the nerve and provided immediate relief. After three weeks her post-operative back pain was gone, and she was able to discontinue her pain medication. Jane started physical therapy about five weeks after surgery and was soon able to return to work. Although her job was physically demanding and required heavy lifting, she could perform her duties if she was careful to lift properly and her co-workers helped out with the heavier loads. She was back on the job full-time within eight weeks.

Jane's story is typical of IA patients: she wasn't under an undue amount of stress, her spinal pathology was clearly seen on the MRI and the pattern of pain was the exact pathway of the 5th lumbar nerve.

Type IB—Structural Source/Hyper-vigilant Nervous System

For patients in the Type IB quadrant, decision-making is more complicated. While an imaging study has identified a structural problem, the patient's nervous system is so sensitized by stress chemicals that their pain is intensified (Chen). If you have identified yourself as a Type IB, consider the following:

- Calming down your nervous system will give you a more accurate perception of your pain and increase your coping capacity. As you reduce your levels of stress hormones, you raise your pain threshold (Chen).

- Your judgment may be impaired when you are frustrated or angry, putting you at a disadvantage when it comes to deciding about surgery.

- Type IB patients frequently resolve their symptoms with non-surgical treatments, even when imaging studies have identified the probable anatomical sources of their pain.

- By systematically addressing all the variables that affect pain, surgical outcomes are more consistent and some patients experience pain relief even without the planned surgery.

As long as you are actively implementing the treatment strategies presented in Chapter 7, it should be okay to proceed with surgery. At a minimum you should be:

- Sleeping at least seven hours through the night (with sleep medications if necessary) for three or four weeks.

- Exercising gently 3 – 4 hours per week

- Lowering anxiety, irritability, and anger levels to less than five on a scale of 1 – 10 (with anti-anxiety medications if necessary)

Maximizing Surgical Outcome with a Structured Care Approach

When Rachel was a teenager, she underwent a fusion for scoliosis that extended from below her neck to her mid-low back. When I saw Rachel at age 50, the fusion had broken down (a common occurrence, especially with a long fusion), constricting nerves and causing back and leg pain. I performed a simple laminectomy just below the fusion between her 4th and 5th vertebra. She did well for about six months—but then her pain returned.

Then I discovered that Rachel was under significant stress. She was perfectionistic and self-critical, she had inadequate conflict resolution and coping skills, and she had major parenting differences with her husband over their two young children. When she opted to have a major front and back fusion she was anxious and depressed. Her narcotic usage was astronomical and she stayed in bed for much of the day. With her husband working sixty hours a week and running the household, the marital conflict intensified.

Clearly, Rachel was a Type IB, and she was now in worse shape than before the operation I had performed. Her latest structural problem was a destabilized spine and narrowing (stenosis) at L4-5. Again, I felt I would be able to help her with surgery, in spite of her stress level.

After extending her fusion to her pelvis so that her whole spine was solidly fused, I was shocked when her pain and function did not improve. She continued to take high doses of narcotics and remain bedridden; her marriage continued to deteriorate.

I applied every strategy of structured rehab I knew: We worked on stress, sleep, medications, counseling, physical therapy, and goal setting. After seeing her two or three times a month for over a year, she was almost completely recovered—nearly fully functional and on minimal medications. Five years later she was still doing well.

In retrospect, it probably would have been better for Rachel to work through structured rehab before undergoing any surgery. The narrowing below her fusion obviously had been there before; but her high stress levels caused it to be symptomatic. I can't be sure if she could have avoided surgery altogether; but by first working with her on non-surgical interventions, months of suffering might have been prevented.

To insure the best possible treatment outcome, calm down your nervous system. You have no way of knowing if your pain will improve *without* surgery until you do. There are obvious exceptions: If a structural problem is so severe as to be causing crippling pain or neurological deficits, such as widespread weakness, foot drop, bicep weakness, etc., your surgeon might want to proceed quickly with the operation, regardless of your stress level.

Type IIA—Non-structural/Calm

As a Type IIA patient, you are a relatively calm person with good coping skills. Your imaging study did not reveal an anatomical reason for your pain, but you are open to non-surgical rehab strategies. Although your discomfort may be fairly unpleasant at times, you are handling it reasonably well, even to the point of being able to tolerate uncomfortable soft-tissue manipulations.

Type IIA patients rarely undergo surgery and don't push for it. Even during the first ten years of my practice when I was relatively aggressive about performing fusions for low back pain—once I explained the nature of the surgery, the risks, and the expected outcome, Type IIA patients tended to opt out. Weighing the uncertainty and the magnitude of surgery, they decided it wasn't worth the risk.

The treatment path for those in the Type IIA quadrant is generally education, medications, and physical therapy. Additional non-surgical approaches that can contribute to your treatment include massage, weight training, yoga, Feldenkrais, Tai Chi, acupuncture and chiropractic care, among many others.

Those in the Type IIA group should avoid surgery under any circumstances. Why would you undergo a risky, unpredictable operation on your perfectly functional spine when there is no visible structural problem other than, possibly, age-related conditions that are normal and rarely cause pain; you are active; and you have many effective non-surgical treatment options available to you?

Unfortunately, medical professionals have convinced many Type IIA patients that they should have spine surgery. The argument goes like this: "You've been in pain for more than three months and none of the other treatment methods worked." In doctor-speak, you have failed conservative care. You are also the ideal surgical candidate, because you are well-adjusted, motivated, and "will do well with surgery."

Type IIA's do well *without* surgery. There should not be a flicker of doubt about just saying "no" to a surgeon who recommends a procedure. However, if your pain doesn't abate after a few weeks of rehab, your surgeon may do well to revisit other pain sources and reassess the role of stress.

Successful Non-surgical Treatment of Spondylolisthesis

Tom was a 29-year-old executive who had been experiencing low back pain for over year. He had a condition at L5-S1 called isthmic spondylolisthesis, a bony defect at the back of the spine that allows a vertebra to slip forward onto the one below. His disc was otherwise normal, and there was only minimal slippage. He did not have excessive motion as measured by bending backwards and forwards, so it was stable. With only axial pain and no instability, Tom's pain source was Type II, non-structural.

Tom was in excellent physical condition; and although his discomfort wasn't debilitating, it frustrated him when the pain limited his tennis and jogging. He was working full time in sales, with the usual stresses that come with the territory, and was engaged to be married. In short, Tom was coping well in spite of his pain, with a reasonably calm nervous system: a classic IIA patient.

After two surgeons had recommended a fusion at the level of his spondylolisthesis, Tom saw me for another opinion. I hadn't the faintest inclination toward an operation. Instead, I recommended that Tom switch to a physical therapist who would pay more attention to his posture, body mechanics, and stretching of the muscles around his hips. I convinced him to return to a weight-lifting regimen in the gym and tuned up his sleep habits. His pain resolved in about six weeks, and three years later he had no pain or physical limitations.

Tom's situation was typical of many patients with spondylolisthesis and back pain. There is a strong mindset among surgeons to perform fusions for this condition; but there is no evidence that it is the source of pain, especially when the spine is stable.

I have seen many IIA patients unnecessarily fused for back pain, opening up opportunities for complications, future surgeries, and increased pain. Non-surgical treatment of a Type IIA is consistently successful, when combined with thoughtful attention to detail and the patient's sincere engagement in the treatment activities.

Type IIB—Non-structural/Hyper-vigilant Nervous System

If you identify with Type IIB, you need to take extra care. With the combination of high stress levels and relentless pain with no clear structural explanation, you might be tempted to opt for surgery on the off chance that it will end your misery. But in fact the opposite is true. While your group ends up having the most surgeries, it also has the least successful outcomes (Nguyen, Franklin).

Of all the groups on the grid, IIBs are the most vulnerable. Although their surgeons explain the risks of surgery, IIBs may be unable to understand and internalize the prospect of a failed surgery, so intent are they to escape their misery. But when surgery fails, Type IIB patients are left not only with their pre-existing problems; they have *increased* pain and a spine that's more structurally damaged.

My message to Type IIB patients is: Don't agree to an operation, even if you are at the end of your rope. Instead, the best course of treatment for you, with the greatest likelihood of success, is an extensive structured rehab program. It takes patience and commitment, which I understand may be in short supply right now; But there is nothing to lose with a structured rehab program except your anxiety, fatigue, depression, and your chronic pain.

Even IB patients with identifiable surgical lesions have unpredictable outcomes if they don't learn the practices that will decrease their levels of stress hormones. Similar to the IB group who needs to move into the IA group before surgery, your goal is to become a Type IIA patient. Learning that there is no visible problem to account for your pain can be overwhelming, leaving you feeling hopeless. I strongly suggest the following:

- Engage fully in an organized structured rehab program that addresses every aspect of chronic pain—physical, emotional, and behavioral. You could employ a self-directed program such as the one in my book, *Back in Control: A Surgeon's Roadmap Out of Chronic Pain,* 2nd edition, or any other book, clinic, or system you prefer.

- Keep in mind that 5% of patients are responsible for 55% of health-care dollars spent in the United States, and Type IIB patients figure prominently in that 5%. The pursuit of pain relief in the form of unfounded surgery is exorbitantly expensive (Lieberman).

- Give yourself a pat on the back. Many Type IIB patients wouldn't even consider reading a book like this or take the initiative to explore new points of view to resolve their pain. You've already astronomically increased your chances of winning the battle.

Failed Surgery in a IIB Patient

Mary, a middle-aged mother of two young boys, sought treatment for low back pain, barely able to get around with a walker. She had been physically inactive for a couple of years and gained a lot weight; also, her marriage was in trouble.

Mary had a small but stable degree of scoliosis—not a source of pain. I felt that surgery wasn't even a remote choice, and recommended a comprehensive rehab program. She did not care for my opinion, and found another surgeon who would perform surgery. He fused the lowest four levels of her spine, requiring the insertion of a metal rod to stabilize the spine while the fusion became solid, a process that usually takes 4 - 6 months.

About six months after Mary's operation, her back broke above the fusion, and her spine now tilted forward about sixty degrees. When she saw me, she was doubled over in a wheelchair, with painful sores on her buttocks. Her husband had left her and their two children, and she was so emotional that we were barely able to have a conversation. She now had moved into the IB quadrant with severe structural problems, all caused by her ill-advised surgery.

I never could calm Mary down enough to discuss the next steps of her treatment (corrective surgery combined with structured rehab). She never returned.

Summary

The Treatment Grid gives you a treatment pathway specific to your situation. Make sure you are in the correct quadrant in the Treatment Grid. Being in the correct quadrant will eventually yield a consistently effective treatment approach. Being in the wrong quadrant can have devastating results.

CHAPTER 6

Understanding Chronic Pain

THERE HAS BEEN A LOT OF CONTROVERSY around the treatment of chronic pain, and patients and physicians alike are frustrated by the inability to solve it. Chronic pain is a complicated phenomenon shaped by many influences, and modern medicine's approach is to offer simplistic, random solutions while ignoring current neuroscience that points the way to a new paradigm. The current definition of chronic pain is "...an embedded memory that becomes associated with more and more life experiences, and the memory cannot be erased" (Mansour). This chapter will explain how this process evolves and why understanding the neurochemical nature of chronic pain is the first step to resolving it.

Most surgeons and patients take for granted that pain is the result of damage to the body, and if that damage can be repaired, the pain will resolve. This mechanistic approach is not out of line with what I have argued—that pain caused by identifiable sources can be pursued with surgery. After all, when you take your car into the shop and have a faulty part repaired or replaced, it usually solves the problem, providing the mechanic made a correct diagnosis. When you drive it out of the shop, the car feels as good as new.

However, people are not machines. For one thing, machines do not experience pain. They do not have nervous systems, emotions, hormones, or memories—all of which, among other things, greatly affect pain perception. There are an estimated 85 billion neurons in your brain and at least at many glial cells providing support to the neurons (Lent). The neurons connect to each other in a multitude of ways, yielding an almost infinite number of combinations. Your soft tissues contain about a million pain receptors per square inch. Through the peripheral and autonomic nervous systems, almost every cell in your body is intertwined with the central processing unit we call the brain. No machine can ever match this complexity.

Why is it Important to Assess the State of My Nervous System?

Let's consider another man-made machine, much more complex than a car. A Boeing 747 jetliner has over two million components, each precisely engineered to safely transport 300 tons of cargo. Coordinating all these components is a complex computer system, the "mind" of the jet. Thus the "body" and "mind" of the vessel are interdependent, working together every second that the jet is in use. One is useless without the other.

So it is with you. Your mind and body are constantly working together around the clock—except that, instead of two million components like the jet, trillions of parts carry out your functions, satisfy your needs, and keep you alive. To these ends, you gather information from the environment, process it, and appropriately act or react. Your unconscious brain at any moment processes a million times more bits of information than does the conscious brain (Trinker).

As environmental input bombards your sensory receptors, it travels through your peripheral and autonomic nervous systems to your central nervous system (brain and spinal cord), where it is immediately analyzed: Is the stimulus pleasant or unpleasant? Safe or dangerous? Your brain then automatically directs your behavior to keep you safe. This complex, protective scheme is called the nociceptive system.

For example, the sensors in your eyes, in the form of rods and cones, send impulses to your brain through the optic nerve, which sends back signals to dilate or constrict your pupils, depending on the level of brightness your sensors detect. You'll instinctively look away from the sun to protect your eyes. Taste receptors quickly detect potentially poisonous substances. Pressure sensors cause you to shift in your chair to avoid skin breakdown. People who are paralyzed, lacking pain receptors below the level of injury, develop skin sores and deep ulcers if they do not manually shift their positions periodically.

The nociceptive system keeps us safe—and alive. None of your sensory receptors by itself has the ability to recognize a threat or a benefit. For that, every bit of sensory input must be analyzed by the central nervous system. Like the airliner with its computer and copious components, there is no separation between mind and body. Together, the two form an interdependent unit.

Survival

Our sensations of pleasure and pain allow us to survive and evolve by guiding us away from danger and toward food, shelter, safety, community, and mates. Pain is part of a wonderfully delicate and complex feedback system designed to protect you. People who are born without the ability to feel pain, a rare condition called *congenital indifference to pain*, rarely survive beyond age ten because, without pain stimuli, they cannot learn how protect themselves. They perish from repeated infections in traumatized tissues (Brand).

A laboratory experiment that measured the amount of pain reported by volunteer subjects dramatically demonstrated the extent to which the brain takes into account all input. When the experimenters introduced a visual stimulus with the pain, they found that those subjects who watched a red light reported perceiving more pain than those who watched a blue one (Moseley).

Since pain signals injury to the body, we naturally take steps to eliminate it, either consciously or unconsciously; and most of the time we're successful. Once we take action and eliminate a pain sensation, we have taken ourselves out of danger. But then how do we explain the persistence of pain after we have gotten rid of the offending stimulus or the inflamed, irritated tissues have healed? The answer may lie in what I call "The Curse of Consciousness."

The Curse of Consciousness

The Curse of Consciousness is humans' inability to escape from thoughts. What does this have to do with chronic pain? Mental pain (unpleasant thoughts) creates a similar bodily reaction as physical pain; but, whereas our nociceptive system allows us to quickly escape from physical pain, we lack an automatic protection system to escape from mental or emotional pain. As this is a universal problem, we are all subjected to varying degrees of chronic stress and fluctuating levels of stress hormones (Eisenberger).

Say you are remembering the attractive person you met last night. That thought triggers the secretion of oxytocin, the bonding love-drug. You recall, in fact, that the whole evening was charming, and you produce some dopamine, the pleasure and reward hormone. As you smile, serotonin, an anti-depressant, enters your bloodstream, and gamma-Aminobutyric acid (GABA) elicits the relaxation response. Thanks to all these pleasure-inducing chemicals, you feel happy. Perhaps you start planning a way to repeat the experience.

Conversely, unpleasant thoughts will trigger the manufacture of the "fight-or-flight" hormones adrenaline, cortisol, and norepinephrine. Suppose you see an email in your inbox from the IRS or from your ex-spouse. Your blood pressure begins to rise and your breathing becomes shallow. You don't even know what the message says yet; it's only an email. All the same, your brain goes into high alert and your body reacts. Whether your thoughts are rational or fantastical, the stress chemicals are released.

Try not to think of a white elephant. It is well documented that when you try to suppress a thought, you'll think about it more. A famous 1987 Harvard paper known as the "White Bears Experiment" (Wegener), demonstrated that subjects who were told to avoid thinking about something—in this case, a white bear—thought about it more frequently than subjects who were told to think about anything they liked. The reverse is also true: If you try to think about something more, you'll think about it less.

This is not good news for chronic pain sufferers. Because we process unpleasant repetitive thoughts (URTs) in a similar region of the brain as physical threats, we trigger stress hormones just with our thoughts. Trying to suppress or mask URTs only increases their recurrence. As we'll see below, the resulting chemical environment causes many diverse physical symptoms.

If that news isn't bad enough, your highly efficient brain embeds your thoughts in memory the same way it does your physical reality (Barrett). This allows us to build on experiences in our environment, so that we don't need to keep learning the same lessons over and over. You recognize a chair when you see one because your brain has unscrambled the visual signals from past experience. Your belief systems—and pain—are established the same way.

The Evolution of Chronic Pain

The brain is a dynamic structure, changing every millisecond. New nerve cells are formed, additional connections through small tentacles called *dendrites* are created, myelin (the insulation around the nerves) thickens and thins, and glial cells (supporting structural cells) undergo ongoing revision. The constantly changing nature of the brain, called *neuroplasticity*, allows us to learn and adapt quickly.

In order to understand how you came to develop chronic pain, we need to consider these ongoing changes within the nervous system. In addition to the chemical effects we have already discussed, three other factors contribute to the development of chronic pain. They are:

- Sensitization

- Memorization

- The "modifiers"— anxiety, anger, and sleep

Sensitization

I have encountered scores of patients who strongly believed that, if their chronic pain got worse, some anatomical problem was progressing—even in the absence of further injury. Actually, in most cases the pain worsens simply because of the way the brain processes repetitive stimuli.

When your brain is constantly bombarded with pain impulses, it will eventually take less of an impulse to elicit the same response (pain) in the brain. In addition, that same impulse can cause more neurons in the brain to fire, resulting in patients complaining that their pain is getting worse although there is no additional trauma. They have become sensitized to their pain.

This phenomenon was clearly documented in a clinical study performed in 2004 (Giesecke). As pain-free volunteers had light pressure applied to one of their fingers, the researchers measured the response in their brains with a functional magnetic resonance imaging machine (fMRI), which tracks metabolic activity. Researchers consistently identified only one small area of the brain that responded to the pressure. They then applied the same pressure stimulus to patients who were experiencing chronic pain. There were two chronic pain groups: one consisted of people with chronic lower-back pain (CLBP) of more than three months; the other consisted of people who suffered from fibromyalgia (chronically widespread musculoskeletal pain). In both groups, five areas of the brain lit up. Although the fibromyalgia group experienced more diffuse body pain, anxiety, and depression than the CLBP group, the fMRI scan data were almost identical.

Memorization

Memorized Pain

Another consequence of repetition of pain impulses is memorization. When pain impulses are repeated for any length of time, the brain "learns" them. However, while it might take years to become an expert baseball player or pianist, pain can be memorized within a matter of months. Once learned, the memory is permanent—just like riding a bicycle.

A prime example of memorization is the "phantom limb" phenomenon, which occurs in patients who have had a limb amputated after experiencing great pain from disease or trauma. After the limb is removed, up to 60% of patients still feel pain, as though the limb were still there. Almost 40% of sufferers characterize the pain as anywhere from distressing to even more severe than before (Gallagher). The neurological connections associated with pain continue to function, even when the offending stimulus is removed.

Memorized Thoughts

As we discussed earlier in this chapter, "the curse of consciousness" may be the biggest culprit in creating chronic pain. As your brain memorizes unpleasant thoughts, they can develop into uncontrollable, obsessive loops. Hard as you try to make them go away, repressing them actually gives negative thoughts more neurological attention. "The surgeon screwed up my back." "I can't get out of bed." "The pain is ruining my life." If left unchecked, recurring thoughts can become stubborn obstacles to recovery.

Strangely, the more legitimate your complaints, the more havoc they create. Maybe you are right. Maybe the surgeon did screw up your back. Maybe you really can't get out of bed without help. And that makes it all the more difficult to let those thoughts go.

And what about the physical manifestations brought on by your repetitive, unsettling thoughts and the feelings they generate? Your bodily reactions, including your chronic pain, are manifestations of the body's stress hormones and intimately tied to your thought-generated negative stimuli.

One landmark study compared fMRIs of volunteers suffering from acute low back pain (less than two months) to those with chronic LBP (over ten years), and recorded the areas of the brain that "lit up" during pain sensations. The acute group's brain activity was confined to the area known for low back pain; while the chronic group's activity was located in the emotional centers of the brain (Hashmi). The experimenters then followed a subset of acute patients for a year. In the subjects whose pain became chronic, the brain activity shifted from the areas associated with acute back pain to the emotional centers. In the group whose symptoms resolved, both areas quieted down.

Neurons that fire together wire together. When pain sensations are located in the emotional area of your brain, they can be triggered by unpleasant thoughts.

We each have some version of a negative thought loop. "I'm not good enough." "What will people think?" "How am I going to pay my bills?" "What's wrong with me?" Obsessive thought loops are so common that we think of them as normal. Like phantom limb pain, they haunt us because they have become neurologically embedded. I call them "phantom brain pain."

Phantom Brain Pain as a Body Image Disorder

Early in my career I performed major reconstructive spine surgery on an athletic 27-year-old patient. Brad had a moderate "hunchback" from a deformity called *kyphosis*, which he felt was causing him thoracic pain. Brad's back tilted forward about 80 degrees, where "normal" is considered no more than 55 degrees. I was hesitant to perform surgery, as it was a 5 – 6-hour procedure with significant risks. But the operation went well and reduced Brad's kyphosis to below 50 degrees, well within normal range. The procedure, however, altered neither Brad's pain nor his body image. He was still obsessed with the shape of his spine and could not appreciate the significant correction we achieved under great risk. It seemed like a classic case of "phantom brain pain." After years of emotional and physical pain triggered by his spine deformity, he continued to suffer even after the problem had been remedied.

Regardless of the origins of your chronic pain, repetitive pain signals bombard your brain and form lasting memories. Knowing this, it is imperative that you visualize your pain as a network of well established, programmed circuits. You can never remove or "fix" these neural connections by surgery or any other means. But by using re-programming tools, you can create pain-free "detours" around old pain circuits. We will explore several tried-and-true methods in Chapter 7.

The Modifiers: Anxiety, Anger, and Sleep

As memorized pain circuits and negative thought loops sensitize your nervous system, both physical and emotional pain intensifies. Your body, ever vigilant to protect you, responds with more stress chemicals, inviting anxiety, anger, and sleeplessness to the party.

Other physical symptoms can appear during hyper-alert states as well. The combination of sleep deprivation, chronic anxiety, and anxiety-fueled anger can become intolerable—for both you and those close to you.

Anxiety

Anxiety is not a diagnosis; it is a symptom. Anxiety is that deeply unpleasant sensation that signals the presence of elevated levels of stress hormones, which you generated in response to a threat. Whether the threat is a physical reality or a negative thought, the body's response is the same. The unpleasant sensation is there to compel you to resolve the problem, to survive.

What if the threat is habitual self-doubt, recurring thoughts such as "I'm not good enough" or "I'm not attractive"? Since such sources of anxiety are not readily solvable, you suffer sustained levels of stress hormones that wreak havoc on your body. Your efforts to ignore these thoughts, suppress them, or distract yourself are not only futile, but actually increase the levels of these chemicals. The long-term consequence of chronic stress is a life expectancy of seven years less than the average population (Torrance). Other punishing effects on your body include:

- Increased blood supply to your muscles and skin, causing tension and perspiration

- Decreased blood flow to your intestines and bladder, causing irritable bowel syndrome and spastic bladder

- Accelerated nerve conduction, resulting in heightened pain sensitivity

- Persistent state of alert, causing fear and emotional hypersensitivity

- Heart palpitations

- Compromised immune system, increasing vulnerability to disease and autoimmune disorders

- Altered blood flow to your brain, increasing susceptibility to migraines

- Changes in breathing patterns, triggering shortness of breath and asthma attacks

More bodily manifestations of anxiety are listed in Chapter 4.

Since anxiety is part of your unconscious survival mechanism, it is largely outside your realm of control, unaffected by rational intervention. For most people, unrelenting anxiety is the worst part of chronic pain. They feel trapped in a deep, dark pit of despair, a place I call the "Abyss."

Anger

As far as your nervous system is concerned, anxiety and anger are one and the same. Like anxiety, anger is generated by high levels of stress chemicals. As one of your body's responses to regain control, it is ironic that anger often puts you even more out of control.

There is a "genealogy" of anger:

1. Anger-provoking situation (real or imagined)

2. Blame

3. Victim role

4. Anger

Examples of anger-inducing situations include:

-   Invasion of your boundaries by
    -   Your boss
    -   A bully
    -   Your spouse
-   Inability to meet your basic physical needs for
    -   Food
    -   Water
    -   Air
    -   Shelter
    -   Comfort
-   Inability to meet your basic psychological needs for
    -   Love and acceptance

- Security
- Acknowledgment and recognition
- Peace

If the extra chemical kick provided by your anger allows you to solve the problem, your anger will abate. If not, the levels of stress hormones go even higher, causing more intense and frequent physical reactions. The late Dr. John Sarno, a prominent rehab physician and author, aptly used the word, "rage" to describe this state of existence when trapped by pain. Pain is just one item of a long list of stimuli that incite anger. Some others include:

- A chaotic relationship or household

- Dependency on disability benefits

- Financial deficits, especially if basic needs like food and shelter are compromised

- Being endlessly bounced around the medical system.

- Traffic

- Work situation, such as a difficult supervisor or co-worker

You get the idea. Anger is destructive because it is focused only on *your* survival. Relationships are particularly affected. The more intimate the relationship, the worse the damage. Instead of cultivating much-needed family support, the angry chronic pain patient often targets his or her family with verbal, emotional or physical abuse. Destructive tendencies also turn inward. One manifestation is complete disregard for one's health. Another that many patients fall into is deep depression and hopelessness. However, all these symptoms abate, when you can let go of your anger. It is a learned skill.

Sleep

Addressing sleep disorders is the first step towards the resolution of chronic pain. Adequate sleep is necessary for processing, organizing, and de-cluttering information taken in by your brain during the day. Loss of even one night's rest impairs judgment, learning, and response times. But sleep deprivation also profoundly affects chronic pain. The research literature is rich with studies about the relationship of sleep and pain.

Insomnia seems to be associated with a higher intensity of pain (Karaman). Sleep deprivation for just one night lowers the pain threshold (Onen). One study, which followed more than 2,000 patients for almost four years, found that people with insomnia have nearly a 40% higher chance of suffering from chronic back pain (Agmon). While this study did not find evidence of the reverse relationship (Pain suffering did not lead to poor sleep), other studies have.

A large survey performed in Turkey found that patients in chronic pain had almost double the insomnia compared to those without pain. Another study, which surveyed around 19,000 individuals from five European countries, showed that people with chronically painful conditions (e.g., limb or joint pain, backache, gastrointestinal pain, headache) experienced significantly more insomnia than those without pain. Compared to individuals without chronic pain conditions, those with pain were three times more likely to report difficulties with initiating sleep, maintaining sleep, early morning awakenings, and non-restorative sleep (Ohayon).

In addition to aggravating your pain and compromising your capacity to cope, sleep deprivation interferes with thinking clearly, which may affect your ability to make sound decisions about your care. Prior to considering surgery you should be sleeping at least six cumulative (but not necessarily consecutive) hours during a 24-hour period for a minimum of six weeks. Insomnia is treatable with minimal risks.

Summary

Chronic pain is a complex neurochemical response that becomes embedded in the nervous system. Mental pain is processed in a similar manner as physical pain; but since we can't escape our thoughts, we are subjected to sustained, elevated levels of stress hormones. As this is part of the unconscious brain, it is not responsive to rational interventions.

Factors that contribute to the development of chronic pain are 1) neural sensitization, 2) memorization of pain circuits, and 3) the modifiers anxiety, anger, and sleep. To effectively treat chronic pain, you must first understand its nature. By addressing all aspects of it, chronic pain is a solvable problem.

CHAPTER 7

Resolving Chronic Pain

As you begin your healing journey, you may find yourself facing one of the following dilemmas:

- Surgery is an option. Is it possible to avoid surgery and resolve my pain?
- Surgery is the best choice for me. How can I optimize the result?
- Surgery was successful, but my symptoms returned. Now what do I do?
- Surgery was unsuccessful. What should I do?
- Surgery is not a choice. Do I have any other options?

The essence of resolving chronic pain is connecting to your own healing power through your ability to regulate your body's chemistry. This chapter introduces you to tools that are crucial to your healing, whether or not surgery is part of your solution. By moving from a Type B, sensitized nervous system into the Type A, calm group, you will be on your way to solving your chronic pain.

Anxiety: The Substance of Chronic Pain

Relentless anxiety is a danger sign that stress hormones are bathing every cell in your body. After exhibiting a variety of physical symptoms, your body eventually will break down and become sick. You may even face early death (Torrance). The saying "Stress kills" is not to be taken lightly, especially if you are considering an operation. You need to calm down your nervous system before you embark on the additional stress of major surgery. Consider the following progression of anxiety levels:

- Alert
- Nervous
- Afraid
- Panicked
- Paranoid
- Terrorized

Every living creature on this planet endeavors to survive by avoiding threats and seeking rewards. We wouldn't have survived without anxiety: It has evolved to be unpleasant, compelling us to take action. But when the situation prevents us from taking action, we feel trapped and miserable—unless we learn how to lower our levels of stress hormones. Since anxiety is a symptom of elevated stress chemicals, once we learn how to control the levels of these chemicals, we will have control over our anxiety, rather than it controlling us.

Solution Principles: Solving the Unsolvable

By understanding that anxiety is only feedback about the state of your body, you can detach from it rather than identify with it. Putting it another way, you can observe it rather than trying to avoid it. It is an important step. Compare it to the engine's temperature gauge in your car: The more you feel threatened, whether the threat is real or imagined, the higher the reading on your anxiety gauge. But, as the temperature gauge in your car does not represent your whole car or even your whole engine (only its temperature); your anxiety does not define you or your life—it's only a measure of your stress-hormone level. You can read it objectively and take appropriate action when it rises to uncomfortable levels. These actions consist of techniques to lower your stress chemicals—both directly, by employing relaxation techniques; and indirectly, by reducing your brain's reactivity.

Direct Approach: Employ Relaxation Techniques

Relaxation techniques reduce the stress response and strengthen the relaxation response, resulting in a body chemistry that is less sensitive to pain and more conducive to better treatment outcomes. Such practices as taking long, deep breaths; meditating; doing yoga or tai chi; walking in nature; guided imagery; and body scan (progressive muscle relaxation) are a few popular methods.

Direct approaches are ideal for addressing day-to-day, minute-to-minute reactions to stress. A favorite of mine is *active meditation.* When you feel anxious or upset, simply focus on a physical sensation such as touch, sight, sound, etc. for five to ten seconds. You can do this as many times a day as needed. Over time, it becomes fairly automatic.

Another direct strategy is reminding yourself that any time you are anxious or upset, you have been triggered. In other words, a current situation has reminded you of an unpleasant experience from the past and your brain says "Danger!" When you are triggered, your unconscious brain takes over your rational thinking, and you may behave badly or make poor decisions. In these situations, it is wise to withdraw from the triggering incident until the energy spike has abated. A mantra I have found helpful is "No action in reaction." Use whatever method you find most effective.

Indirect Approach: Harness your Brain's Neuroplasticity

The complexity of the brain is beyond our comprehension. But we do know that we can rewire our brains by creating "detours" around pre-existing pain circuits. The process is similar to an athlete or musician learning a skill with repetition: New circuits are created and strengthened. However, if you try to *eliminate* unpleasant pathways, you will place neurological attention on them, reinforcing them.

Consider another example, that of learning a new language. To master a foreign language requires a focused commitment for a long period of time. Eventually, you will have developed a new part of your brain that enables you to speak the new language. You will have increased the number of neurons and connections between them, laid down new insulating material (*myelin*), and brought about changes in the supporting *glial cells.* This is the essence of neuroplasticity (Dragananski).

Your brain never stops adapting and reprogramming. Why not encourage neuroplastic changes to your benefit? For example, you can "rewire" your brain to be less reactive to triggers that spike your reactivity.

Instead of the normal scenario, which usually goes:
Threat > Automatic survival response
You can change it to:
Threat > Chosen response

You first feel the emotion, create some "space" for an instant, and then substitute a more desirable response. You can create this space using such techniques as writing down your feelings, practicing awareness of your automatic reactions, taking a deep breath, and so on. The key is to avoid immediately reacting to something that is upsetting or anxiety-producing. The sequence is *awareness, detachment, reprogramming.* It works. The result is less frequent reactivity, shorter chemical surges, and lower anxiety.

You obviously can't learn a foreign language by merely avoiding your native language or trying to improve on it. Neither can you solve chronic pain by working on it or trying to avoid it. Where is your attention? What circuits are you reinforcing? By constantly (understandably) seeking a cure or discussing your pain with those around you, you reinforce your pain circuits. As they become more deeply embedded in your nervous system, they become more difficult to extinguish. You also limit your creative activity. Research shows that the brain physically shrinks in the presence of chronic pain—although fortunately it re-expands when you have healed. (Apkarian).

The best course of action is to learn a "new language" called "an enjoyable life." Anxiety and anger are hard-wired, primitive survival responses, and they become stronger with age and repetition. Retraining your brain requires deliberate, long-term, focused effort.

The first step in any new endeavor is to visualize your destination. What do you want your life to look like? What do you want to leave behind? When you pursue a desired goal, you expand your nervous system. As you learn the new language called "an enjoyable life" and pay less attention to old pain circuits, the neglected circuits will recede from disuse.

At some point your pain and anxiety will diminish dramatically—but not by *resisting* it. The process is similar to re-directing a river to a new channel. It may be slow at first; but as the water is diverted, it will create the new passage.

Take Action

A serious effort to reduce or eliminate chronic pain must contain the following three components, all of which contribute to modifying your body's chemical makeup.

- Awareness
    - Of your diagnosis
    - Of all treatment options
    - Of your pain and your relationship to it
- Simultaneous treatment of all components of your pain experience
- Taking charge of your own care

Awareness

Thoughtful study is a necessary step for any problem-solving task. You would never walk into an architectural firm and demand, merely, "I want a house," expecting to be satisfied with the result. To optimize your chances of a satisfactory outcome, you would spend hours with your architect, researching, planning, designing, and modifying, before any ground was broken.

It makes even less sense to walk into a clinic and say, "I want to be fixed." If a surgeon recommends elective surgery for pain on your initial evaluation after a brief visit, you should walk out.

Obviously, there are exceptions for emergency situations. But I can't begin to describe the misery of patients who have undergone failed spine surgeries and are much worse off than they were before their operation. This is anything but a snap decision. Your surgeon needs to get to know you, and you need to know how to optimize your outcome of treatment, with or without surgery. Your decision will impact the rest of your life.

So, the first step in deciding whether to undergo surgery is developing a working relationship with your surgeon, where all your concerns and issues are fully addressed before a making a final decision. My protocol was to spend at least *three months* with each patient, working towards understanding each other and addressing all the factors that affected that person's perception of pain. On spinal deformity cases, which required especially high-risk operations, I would work with my patients for many months—sometimes years. I proceeded in this manner to avoid contributing to the dismal statistics: 19% of patients undergoing deformity corrections return to the operating room within two years to revise or repair the original surgery; and 7% have multiple return trips to the OR (Kerezoudis).

Complete knowledge of your diagnosis and how it relates to the neurochemical basis of chronic pain is critical. Reading this book will give you the foundations you need; but you still must spend time with your surgeon discussing your choices before you truly understand them. A major component of healing is feeling safe, and that includes your interactions with your physician and the whole surgical team. Don't accept anything less than a thorough understanding of your situation, your options, and the resources available to you.

In addition to your knowledge of your diagnosis and treatment options, you also need to be aware of your relationship to pain. To reroute your nervous system, you have to first know what is going on. This is probably the most challenging aspect of healing: You need to allow yourself to feel and be with your anxiety and frustration as you lay down alternate brain circuits that will circumvent it. Fighting or denying these powerful survival responses only reinforces them.

Simultaneous Treatment of All Components of Your Pain Experience

Chronic pain is a complex problem and all relevant aspects of it must be treated. These are foundational elements to be systematically addressed:

1. **Knowledge:** Understanding the neurological basis of chronic pain
2. **Sleep:** No treatment is effective without adequate sleep.
3. **Stress:** Floods your body with harmful chemicals.
4. **Medications:** Provide symptom relief while you are healing.
5. **Physical conditioning:** Essential to any rehab program for symptom relief, injury prevention, balancing body chemistry, and producing a sense of well-being.
6. **Life outlook:** Shifting your focus from "a life of pain" to "a life well lived" creates a massive nervous system shift from pain circuits to pleasure circuits.

1. Knowledge

Throughout this book, I point out the connection between pain and the state of your nervous system, particularly your levels of stress or pleasure hormones flooding your system. Chapter 6 focuses on the nature of chronic pain, with an emphasis on the role anxiety plays.

2. Sleep

You can no longer ignore the importance of consistent, quality sleep. Sleep deprivation will not only increase your perception of pain; it will also compromise your coping skills and judgment. One large study showed that lack of consistent sleep *induced* chronic lower back pain (Agmon). Because consistent sleep is necessary for the rest of the treatments to be effective, sleep issues must be addressed first. Be sure your doctor knows your sleep habits. There is a wealth of approaches to choose from, for establishing a healthy routine.

3. Stress

In my book, *Back in Control: A Surgeon's Roadmap Out of Chronic Pain* (Hanscom), I present a systematic, self-directed process to solving chronic pain. The process is called Direct your Own Care (DOC), and it consists of tools to calm and reprogram your nervous system. The tools are based on somatic methods that connect thoughts to physical sensations. Some of the practices have been around for centuries; but many lay hidden under today's information overload and hectic pace.

Another approach to reprogramming anxiety-producing neural pathways is to reactivate existing, *enjoyable* circuits that have gotten buried by life situations and pain. Play is important in every person's development, and reconnecting with playfulness is powerful (Brown). Results are swift, and repetition can strengthen pleasurable circuits until they become habitual. When this happens, your body experiences a profound shift from stress chemicals to relaxation hormones. As your organs luxuriate in this rejuvenating chemical bath, your physical symptoms, including your pain, resolve.

4. Medications

Although chronic pain does not cause structural damage, it does reinforce neurological circuits, which makes the pain sensation more difficult to eradicate. Therefore, it is important to get quick and effective symptomatic relief that will address problematic sleep, pain, and anxiety. As the nervous system calms down, the need for medication disappears. The goal, to go pain-free with minimal or no medications, is achievable most of the time, even in patients who have been on high-dose medications for years.

5. Physical Conditioning

Tight muscles and joint contractures are painful. As the injured area approaches full range of motion, your body warns you with pain signals. Becoming more protective of these tissues, your pain grows with less motion. As you decrease your level of activity, your weakened body finds it harder to support your spinal column.

It is imperative to work toward full range of motion of all of your painful joints, as well as spending three to five hours a week doing active resistance exercises, such as weight training. Begin with light weights and many repetitions. Some people even find the repetitions a calming influence.

6. Life Outlook

As you address all these elements of chronic pain simultaneously, your focus shifts toward seeking a full and rich life. The alternative— resolving yourself to a lifetime of suffering—may result in social isolation and a downward spiral of depression. Too many of your waking hours will revolve around pain. Your pain pathways will become your masters, swallowing up your living spirit.

Since emotional pain and physical pain are processed in similar areas of the brain, people who are socially isolated often develop chronic pain (Eisenberger). An essential component of the DOC project is meaningful human connection. People naturally heal each other. Reconnecting with friends and family has been a powerful force in moving away from pain. As you broaden your perspective on life, you will regain the best part of you; and then, the sky will be the limit.

Taking Charge of Your Own Care

The idea of taking control of your own healing may sound impossible and overwhelming. Isn't this a medical problem and shouldn't it be relegated to health professionals?

You could compare solving chronic pain to fighting a forest fire: They are both complex situations, fought on many fronts, requiring multiple solutions. Firefighting consists of assessing the situation, containing it, and removing its fuel. Every fire is different, and extinguishing the blaze requires different strategies depending on the fire's unique characteristics—the height of the flames, local terrain, and weather, to name a few. Fire travels more quickly up a steep hillside in dry, windy conditions; compared to the speed of a brush fire on flat ground on a windless, humid night.

During a wildfire, the fire chief sets up the control base and coordinates the operation. You are the most capable "chief" to put out the fire of your chronic pain. You have spent a lifetime getting to know yourself well enough to gain insight into your problem; your doctor has spent only a few hours assessing your situation.

The truth is, taking charge of your own care is probably the single, most effective way to feel better. When you take control of any situation, you decrease anxiety. Once you understand chronic pain, your diagnosis, and the issues that affect your perception of pain, you will take charge and move forward. I have seen it happen consistently, and it is a lot better than being bounced around the medical system without clear answers.

Currently, mainstream medicine approaches chronic pain as a condition to be managed or accommodated, by "helping you live your best life, in spite of the pain." With all the neuroscience research that has provided exciting, revelatory solutions for chronic pain, generalized medical care has neither acknowledged nor adopted these findings (Young). Instead, spine surgery clinics continue to employ random, simplistic solutions to treat your complex problem. We have consistent evidence that many of these treatments, *especially* surgery for lower back pain, are ineffective (Deyo). For those who are willing to step up, participate in their healing and take charge of their lives, the outcomes have been consistently positive and inspiring.

Taking Charge—Pain-free After Firing His Doctors

A couple of years ago, a friend asked me for an opinion about his back. He had pain and numbness down the side of his leg, the distribution of his fifth lumbar nerve root.

Sure enough, his MRI scan revealed a bone spur between the fifth lumbar and first sacral vertebra as it exited his spine, surrounding his fifth lumbar nerve root. I felt surgery might help, but I also thought he might be able to avoid surgery with exercises that flexed his spine and relaxed him. I wasn't convinced that his pain was severe enough to warrant the risks of surgery.

He elected for surgery in Spain, his home country. It helped for a couple of months before the same pain returned. He underwent a second operation about six months later that worsened his pain. It was then that I looked at a new MRI scan and saw that the bone spur was still there. The surgeon had neglected to remove it—twice—because he had worked only in the center of the spine and not far enough to the side, in the foramen where the nerve exited.

After a year of dealing with all of this, my friend told me that he had finally had enough and "fired everyone." No more doctors, medications, or surgery, he said. He decided to take charge and move forward on his own terms. Within a week his pain disappeared; five years later he has no pain and is playing golf several times a week.

Avoiding Surgery in the Presence of a Structural Problem

Even after I began using the DOC program, although it was powerful, I did not think its non-operative, non-invasive treatments could adequately address structural problems. Using a dental analogy, how can you rehab an infected tooth? Until the structural source of the pain was addressed, I could not see rehab progressing, least of all while the patient was in pain. I would aggressively perform the surgery, so we could move on with the rest of the program. I also felt that patients already suffering from chronic pain couldn't tolerate the additional stress of a structural problem. This was all before I fully understood the connection between stress and pain.

Still, some patients wanted to try the DOC activities first. I worked with them for a few months, waiting for the day they told me they were ready for surgery. A few never did, because their pain had disappeared or dropped to a level where they felt they did not need surgery. After over a hundred patients did the same thing, I was convinced that calming the nervous system caused pain thresholds to rise.

Another Surgical Patient Avoiding Surgery

A middle-aged patient was experiencing pain down both her legs in the pattern of the L5 nerve root. She had significant bone spurs touching both nerves; but I also knew that her husband had passed away unexpectedly about a year earlier, which devastated the family. After resisting the DOC program for a long time, she decided to undergo surgery to free up both nerve roots. Having made her decision, she engaged in the DOC program before her operation, to optimize her surgical outcome. At her pre-operative visit about six weeks later, she reported that her leg symptoms had disappeared. We cancelled her surgery, and three years later she has not returned.

In both this and my friend's case study, the patients had structural problems with matching symptoms: a classic surgery scenario. In the first case, had the surgeon correctly freed my friend's L5 nerve root, his pain probably would have disappeared. But the fact that his bone spur was never removed demonstrated that he could have improved just as successfully without surgery. Likewise, in the second case, surgery probably would have helped the patient, but she ended up not needing it. Notice that both patients solved their own problems by engaging and taking charge. That is why my first book (the one that describes the DOC program) is titled *Back in Control.* Every patient I have seen improve has taken full responsibility for their own pain and care.

You might be wondering, "In such cases, why not perform the operation anyway, so they don't have to worry about the problem coming up again?" There are a several reasons. First, even with a successful operation, pain circuits often continue to get "fired up" under stress, even with no recurrence of the structural problem; so, the operation may not eliminate the pain. Second, even the simplest operation has risks. I could write a book of simple operations that went bad. Third, spine surgery (like most surgery) creates scar tissue that can be permanently irritating. You are always better off avoiding surgery.

Overview of the Direct your Own Care (DOC) Healing Process

The basis of solving either emotional or physical chronic pain is connecting to your natural healing power. Through your ability to regulate your body's chemistry, you can reduce your level of stress-produced hormones, whose constant presence causes all kinds of physical and emotional symptoms, including pain. The DOC process provides a structure that enables you to find your own best approach. The process is highly doable, the idea being to stimulate your brain to change. The strategies include:

- Somatic work—connecting thoughts with physical sensations (expressive writing)
- Relaxation tools—active meditation, mindfulness, meditation, visualization
- Understanding and addressing the impact of pain on the family unit
- Listening—instead of re-hashing your own views, which only reinforces them
- Forgiveness—You can't simultaneously move forward and hang on to the past
- Refraining from discussing your pain or medical care with anyone but your health care providers—redirect your attention away from the pain
- Getting enough sleep—at least seven restful hours per night
- Letting go of the past and moving forward, with *or* without your pain
- Identifying triggers that affect symptoms—and dealing with them
- Creating your vision—How do you want your life to look?
- Getting organized—So you can follow through on your vision
- Returning to familiar, fun activities such as art, hobbies, music, dance, sports, etc.
- Spending quality time with family and friends
- Re-learning how to play—the antithesis of anger
- Giving back—a reward in itself

Each of these tools decreases anxiety by reducing your brain's reactivity to mental and physical threats. These and other effective approaches are explored in my book, *Back in Control: A Surgeon's Roadmap Out of Chronic Pain,* 2nd edition.

Optimizing Surgical Outcomes: Prehab

Let's assume you have gone through the decision-making steps and opted for spine surgery. You can improve your chances of a successful outcome by implementing what I call a *prehab* program before your surgery. Prehab is simply an organized rehab program, only before rather than after surgery. In addition to including all the elements of the DOC process mentioned above, prehab addresses other medical and structural issues that can impact the outcome of surgery.

The data supports the fact that all patients should go through prehab before undergoing any elective surgery, regardless of the magnitude of the operation (Schug, Perkins). With larger procedures and higher stakes, the need for prehab is even greater. Much of the following section is based on a paper out of Northwestern Hospital in Chicago, published in 2010 (Halpin). In their paper, the authors present an organized approach to optimizing outcomes for high-risk spine surgery. They define "high-risk" by the following criteria:

- Over six hours of surgery

- Over six levels fused

- Both the front and back of the spine fused

- Significant cardiac, pulmonary, liver, kidney, or cerebral vascular disease

- Patient over eighty years old

- Surgeon's judgment of "high risk"

- Medical doctor's judgment of "high risk"

Following is a list of recommendations for optimizing surgical outcomes:

- **Shared decision-making**
  The surgeon's role is to assess the patient's situation and determine whether surgery is an option. It may take several visits and tests. Surgeons should avoid making a surgical decision on the patient's first visit and should leave the final decision to the one experiencing the pain.

  I used to give my patients a detailed letter to take home, mull over, and weigh the magnitude, risk, and possible benefits of the surgery against their symptoms. After closely examining these factors, only a small percent of patients "had to have an operation." A surprising number decided that the surgery was simply not worth the risk.

- **Expectations**
  The vast majority of patients think that back surgery will solve their axial pain even though surgery rarely helps with back or neck pain. However, with engagement in a structured long-term rehab program, axial pain is also solvable. Make sure your expectations are realistic: Be clear which pain can be relieved by surgery and which cannot.

- **Nutrition**
  Neglecting your nutritional needs compromises many bodily functions, especially your ability to ward off infection. One indicator of your nutritional status is your serum albumin level, which measures your body's protein.

  A Veterans Administration (VA) study demonstrated that low serum albumin was the best predictor of complications— even better than the American Society of Anesthesiologist's risk system, the ASA score. The mortality rate from any major surgery was increased 29X (2900%) if the albumin was 21g/l versus the norm of 46 g/L and the chance of a significant complication increased 6X (600%). If the albumin fell below the normal level of 35g/ml, the risk for deep wound infection increased by 3X (300%).

  A low albumin score can also indicate poor liver function. Make sure your albumin is normal before surgery; it is a simple blood test (Gibbs).

- **Smoking cessation**
  Smoking dramatically decreases the ability of the spine to heal and to establish a solid fusion. It also increases the risk of cardio-pulmonary complications. Most spine centers require patients to stop smoking cigarettes at least six weeks before they are allowed to undergo an elective fusion.

- **Osteoporosis treatment**
Weak bone is a major problem in spine surgery. Performing a successful fusion requires the precise placement of metal screws in the pedicles, where nerves lie closely on either side. With an osteoporotic spine, it is easier to perforate the pedicle and irritate or damage these nerves. The screws can pull out of the bone more easily, causing the whole construct to fall apart. The healing process is problematic as well, since less metabolic activity occurs within bones afflicted with osteoporosis. Finally, there is a higher chance of a fracture around the fusion. Especially in middle-aged and older patients, bone density should be tested before treatment.

- **Medical workup**
All patients with planned complex surgeries should be given a thorough workup of the major organ systems. Sometimes these tests are performed before any surgical decisions are made, in case the exams reveal a serious risk that must be weighed against the benefits of the proposed operation. The areas that should be assessed before surgery and addressed by a specialist if there is a question are:

  - Heart
  - Blood pressure
  - Liver and kidney function
  - Pulmonary (lung) function
  - Diabetes
  - Anemia (low blood counts)

- **Calming the nervous system**
Reducing the level of stress hormones in your body will optimize your chances of a successful surgery, so use the tools recommended in this chapter to move from a Type B (stressed nervous system) to a Type A (calm). After I discovered the adverse effects of a hyper-vigilant nervous system on pain and surgical outcomes, I refused to perform surgery on any patient unwilling to engage with prehab and take full responsibility for his or her care.

Summary

The key to resolving chronic pain is learning to regulate your body chemistry—particularly the production of stress hormones. The goal is to move from Type B (stressed nervous system) to Type A (calm); or, if you are already a Type A, to stay there. Moving from the B group to the A group has several benefits. They include:

- **Focused decision-making:** Many symptoms abate with rehab, allowing you to assess your structural problem more objectively.

- **Higher pain threshold:** Many patients experience pain relief with simple stress-reducing practices, enabling them to avoid surgery even when they have a structural problem.

- **Increased capacity to fully rehabilitate:** Lowering your level of stress chemicals boosts energy and motivation.

- **Avoiding surgery:** There is some chance that calming the nervous system raises the pain threshold and the pain disappears, obviating the need for surgery.

- **Easier post-operative course:** A calmed-down nervous system will reduce your post-op pain.

By engaging in the DOC process, a self-directed program that focuses on six core areas that affect chronic pain and surgical outcomes, you will be able to take control of your own care and heal your pain.

SECTION 3:
AVOID DISASTER

CHAPTER 8

Beware the IB Group: Failed Back Surgery

THE TYPE IB QUADRANT ON THE Treatment Grid is a dangerous place to be. You have a structural problem and you are under a lot of stress. You are anxious either because of your pain, your impending surgery, an upsetting situation in your life, or all of the above. You are at an immediate disadvantage because your hyper-vigilant nervous system can sabotage even the most perfectly executed procedure.

However, you can still have effective surgery if you combine it with a stress-management program—that is, if you calm down enough to move to the IA (structural/calm) category before surgery, thereby maximizing your chances of a successful outcome. But all that is if you *start out* in the IB category; you're in real trouble if you begin in any other quadrant and *move into* the IB group.

This chapter will help you avoid the pitfalls of the IB category. It is helpful to explore the ways you might end up there, and the impact of each scenario on your recovery:

1. **You started as a Type IB**—stressed, with a structural problem. With a little work on reducing your anxiety levels, you could move out of IB and into IA, optimizing your surgical outcomes and possibly even going pain-free without surgery.

2. **You started as a Type IA**—calm, with a structural problem, but moved to IB, because of a failed surgery or from new stressors. Failed spine surgeries are so common that the condition has been given its own name: Failed Back Surgery Syndrome (FBSS).

3. **You started as a Type IIA**—calm, with no visible structural problem, but became a IB because your spine was damaged by unnecessary or ill-informed surgery, your pain is no better, and probably is worse. You are regretful and angry over your decision to have surgery, because you are worse off than before, and there is no going back.

4. **You started as a Type IIB**—stressed, with no visible structural problem, but moved to IB. You have lots of company, because the majority of unnecessary surgeries are performed on IIB patients, with consistently poor outcomes. You never needed an operation, since there was nothing visible to fix; it didn't work; and the surgery was performed while you were in a highly stressed state, which often worsens or induces pain (Schug). Your spine is now surgically damaged, and pain is still a major issue. Your already high stress levels skyrocketed.

The last two scenarios in the above list occur most frequently. As neither of these groups should even be considered for surgery, they should **never** end up as IBs. The tragedy is that all Type II patients—those with non-structural pain sources—could have chosen (or been offered) effective non-surgical rehab options.

1. Beginning as a IB (Structural/Hyper-vigilant CNS)

Many patients start out as IBs. Often their lives are already stressful, when accidents and injuries are most likely to occur. Maybe they haven't been sleeping well or are simply distracted by problems. If you are in the B group, it is always ideal to calm down and work your way into the A category with rehabilitation strategies that we know to be effective.

In addition to your stressful life situations, you are also facing a painful structural problem. It is easy to jump into surgery, especially if you are going through tough times and would welcome a quick fix. However, the data is clear that operating in the presence of a fired-up nervous system, regardless of how clear the surgical indications, can worsen the pain (Schug). I have made this point several times in this book, but it is worth repeating because it is hard to fathom that a well performed, indicated surgery could make you feel worse.

That is why it is critical to combine surgery in the IB group with comprehensive rehab *before surgery* to optimize the outcomes. The ideal is to move into the IA quadrant. But even if you can't completely get there, just starting the process will help. After engaging in a comprehensive rehab program, many IB's cancel scheduled surgeries because their pain has disappeared.

In my first edition of *Back in Control: A Spine Surgeon's Roadmap Out of Chronic Pain,* I recommended that patients suffering from chronic pain with structural problems undergo surgery promptly and do the rehab later. My thinking was that these patients couldn't tolerate the additional pain generated by the abnormal pathology. My surgical practice stayed reasonably busy, until I saw the data showing that failing to address the patient's nervous system before an operation could increase or even induce pain. Our team began asking *all* patients considering elective surgery to engage in the DOC process for 8 - 12 weeks prior to their operations. Over one hundred patients with surgical lesions cancelled surgery because the pain had resolved merely from their participation in the process.

Prehab completely changed the nature of my practice. Between those patients who rejected our approach and went elsewhere for surgery, and those who cancelled surgery because the rehab program had resolved their pain, my rate of surgery dropped to 4.6% of all new patients. This was well below the usual rate (at least 10% in my clinic and higher in other surgical practices).

But what happened next made up for my reduced business. Now that all surgical patients engaged in our prehab program, those who underwent surgery had less post-operative pain, resumed activities that required movement soon, were less upset by flare-ups, had a more consistently positive outcome, and were a delight to work with. Treating patients in chronic pain with or without surgery became the most enjoyable part of my practice.

When patients with clear surgical indications began to opt out of surgery, it all began to make sense. Most of these patients had been living with problems like bone spurs or nerve constrictions for years; but *their symptoms had appeared only recently.* Something had changed—and it was not their anatomy. As we began to ask more careful questions, we found invariably that the patient had been experiencing some new or unusual amount of stress. From a woman whose boyfriend has become physically abusive; to a teenage child committing suicide; to the break-up of a family, and much, much worse—we were dumbfounded by the sheer amount of emotional pain that many of our chronic pain patients were enduring, and keeping it all in, trying to cope with the stress and maintain normal lives, which were anything but normal.

Trauma, whether emotional or physical, signals the body's chemistry to be on high alert. As a result, pain thresholds (tolerance) drop, and symptoms associated with abnormal anatomy such as narrowing around nerves promptly appear.

As we helped our patients work through stressful times and obtain emotional support, their pain would either disappear or drop to a level they didn't think was worth the risk of surgery. Earlier surgery may have helped them; but we had witnessed problems with post-operative pain control so often that we became adamant that they engage in prehab first.

If you are facing a personal or professional crisis while coping with a painful structural spine problem, be careful. You are in the IB group; and unless the spine problem is an emergency, you'll be wiser to use the strategies that move you towards the IA quadrant before considering surgery.

Holding on to His Anger—and His Pain

Alex, a 50-year-old insurance salesman, had undergone a simple laminectomy about four years before I saw him. The surgery did not provide relief, and now he was experiencing severe pain down his left leg. During surgery, I discovered a fractured facet joint over the nerve corresponding to his leg pain. The prior surgeon had removed too much bone and destabilized the segment. A tremendous amount of force had been compressing this nerve for four years. This was a severe Type I structural problem, and his intense anger placed him into the B group.

I surgically remedied the problem. Normally when I rectify this magnitude of pathology, the patient experiences a dramatic decrease in pain and improvement in quality of life—the expected outcome for a Type IA. However, although his leg pain was reduced, Alex had ongoing back pain. Also ongoing was his anger—anger at his first wife, at the prior surgeon, at the driver of the car who caused his injury—and now at me, because I didn't resolve all his pain.

Alex's pain increased until it ultimately encompassed his entire body. There was nothing I could do, even though I tried to calm him down for over a year. He never let go of his anger, and he became increasing belligerent.

It was many cases like Alex's and the insistence of my nurse that drove me to avoid any elective surgery on patients with sensitized, "fired-up" nervous systems. Experience—and the literature—taught me that it doesn't matter what you do surgically; unless you address the neurological component, you may not be able to resolve chronic pain, even in the presence of compelling anatomy.

2. Beginning as a IA (Structural/Calm)

IA patients are typically living functional and full lives before suddenly developing a spine problem that requires surgery. Their prognosis is generally the best of all four Treatment Grid groups, so it is tragic to see a IA patient move into the IB group. There are several ways that someone in the IA group can become a IB patient:

- An indicated surgery has a complication.

- A simple procedure is indicated, but a complex operation is performed.

- The patient's case is being administered by a public disability system.

If you are already in the IB group and the above scenarios occur, your situation is that much worse.

An indicated surgery has a complication.

Complications are unplanned events during surgery that compromise the patient's outcome. There is always the risk of complication, no matter how small or straightforward the procedure.

When I left my spine fellowship, I was determined that I simply was not going to have *any* complications during my surgeries. It seemed to me that all those I witnessed during my training could have been avoided, even though extraordinary technical surgeons committed them. Boy, was I wrong. I discovered that complications could occur during the most minor of surgeries by the most careful of surgeons. Often the smallest detail would initiate a torrent of problems. There are four categories of complications:

1. **Human error**—An unplanned technical move during surgery that injures an important structure. Examples include penetrating the dural sac, cutting a nerve root, perforating a major blood vessel, and misplacing hardware.

2. **Adverse events**—Repercussions of the procedure such as deep wound infections, blood clots in the legs (some traveling to the lungs), excessive bleeding, and blindness.

3. **Medical difficulties**—Attributed to excessive stress of the operation on the body, the long list includes bladder and kidney infections, pneumonia, stroke, heart failure, bowel infarction, and death.

4. **Future problems**—Issues that arise after a period of time, post-surgery. Frequent ones include spine breakdowns adjacent to fusions, opioid dependence, spinal stenosis and increased pain.

Complications are categorized in terms of "minor" and "major."

Minor complications

Complications are considered minor if they are solvable with minimal impact on the patient's care and outcome. However, if you are the patient experiencing one or more of these complications, you may not agree that they are so minor. Common "minor" complications include:

- Pneumonia
- Urinary tract infections
- Superficial wound breakdown, where the skin won't heal
- Temporary increase in nerve pain

Major complications

In contrast, major complications cause large-scale, permanent damage to the patient and may require a more prolonged recovery period than expected. Such developments are devastating to the patient, his or her family, and the surgeon as well. Common major complications include:

- Deep wound infection, requiring multiple surgeries to clean out
- Cerebrospinal fluid leak that can't be stopped
- Damage to a nerve root, with loss of motor function
- Damage to the spinal cord, causing partial or complete paralysis
- Breakdown of the spine above or below a fusion, manifested by severe degeneration, ruptured disc, fracture, deformity, and/or significant neurological deficits
- Excessive post-operative bleeding
- Blindness
- Misplaced screws, causing nerve injury and pain
- Blood clots traveling to the lung
- Extreme intensification of post-operative pain
- Death, from any number of causes

This alarming list represents only a sample of the major complications I have witnessed over my career. Having a serious medical condition such as diabetes, HIV, or heart disease, in addition to that prompting your back surgery, adds to the probability and variety of unplanned, negative outcomes.

Both major and minor complications occur under the most beneficial circumstances, whether the procedure is large or small, simple or complex. No one plans on having a complication, but no one is immune. Even when a patient has a structural problem with corresponding symptoms and the patient is calm, there is no guarantee that surgery will be successful.

An Unnecessarily Large Operation is Performed for a Relatively Small Problem.

Major advances in technology allow us to perform bigger operations, obtain better correction of deformities, and consistently create a solid fusion—procedures I never would have dreamed possible as a spine fellow in 1985. But just because we can perform ever-larger operations doesn't mean we always should. Problems occur more frequently and their impact more severe as the procedure gets larger, with higher blood loss and more time needed under anesthesia to implant the new instrumentation.

There is a disturbing trend to perform complex and prolonged procedures when a simpler solution would suffice. Even if the surgery goes well, long fusions leave patients with a stiff spine, unable to turn their upper body. There is a 35% chance—that's one in three—of the spine breaking down within a couple of years above a fusion, and no one has figured out how to prevent it (Kim). The obvious solution—performing a smaller operation or avoiding surgery altogether—is rarely explored. And the patients continue to suffer from pain, regardless of the bigger operation.

I trained in Minneapolis at one of the original spine centers that pioneered deformity surgery. Most of our patients were referrals from all over the world with problems that were too complex for their local surgeons to solve. My mentors, as superb technical surgeons as they were, still had high complication rates, simply because of the nature of their tasks. However, they had little choice, given their typical patient's condition when they reached our center.

When I moved to my Seattle practice, one of my senior partners followed the principle that it was best to do as little as possible to solve any given problem. As I implemented that approach, I realized that it was the better choice. Occasionally, if the smaller operation would not be enough, we could usually go back and solve the problem with a larger procedure. Not all surgeons live by this philosophy; many proceed directly with a large procedure. The following examples represent a frequent occurrence.

IA to IB—Operation Too Complex

Bob was a middle-aged software engineer who had a mild scoliosis that caused neither back pain nor limitations of any kind. When he began to feel sciatic pain in his right leg, his imaging study revealed two small bone spurs between his fourth and fifth vertebrae. After about eight weeks of pain, Bob elected to undergo surgery. There was an identifiable source of pain that corresponded to his symptoms, and he was cheerfully calm about it; therefore, a Type IA patient by my definition.

A simple, one-level procedure called a decompression would have taken care of Bob's bone spurs. But he was told his scoliosis needed to be corrected as well. He underwent a ten-hour operation that fused his ninth thoracic vertebrae down to his pelvis (nine levels), requiring the placement of twenty screws in his spine. Three of the screws were misplaced, causing injury to some of the nerves in his left leg (the sciatica had been in his *right* leg). Emerging from surgery with a numb and weak left leg, Bob returned to surgery the next day to correct the problem.

About a year later, I saw Bob in my clinic. He suffered from extreme pain in his back and both legs, and still had weakness in his left leg. A new CT scan showed the three screws, still misplaced. They had broken through his backbone and were in direct contact with nerves. Living with so much pain, Bob became mentally unstable and unable to cope with even simple stresses, a condition which understandably impacted his marriage and his work negatively. Bob had started out as a Type IA patient with a simple Type I spinal stenosis. But an unnecessary procedure, the spinal fusion for his benign scoliosis, had turned him into a Type

IB with one of the most severe anatomical problems I have ever encountered.

We performed surgery to remove the screws that were pushing on his nerve roots and repaired a couple of places that had not fused. Two weeks later, spacers were put into the front of his spine to ensure a solid fusion.

Bob was left with a permanently numb leg and a failed marriage. But owing to continued psychological support most of his strength and mental faculties returned. His courage and commitment to remain functional and hold onto his job through a number of additional health issues was an inspiration.

Bob's case of sciatica from bone spurs was a simple anatomical problem (Type I) that could have been resolved with a two-hour, low-risk operation. His scoliosis was balanced and irrelevant to his pain, so did not need to be addressed surgically. The fusion, which was unwarranted, led to severe chronic pain, a ruined marriage, and a nearly ruined life.

You may be thinking that Bob's experience is extreme, unlikely, and rare. But it's a common occurrence. I do not fault a surgeon whose patient develops complications; it is one of the unavoidable risks of spine surgery. However, the larger the operation, the greater the risk; and it is the surgeon's duty to honestly weigh the necessity and potential benefit of an operation against its magnitude.

The patient's case is being administered by a public disability system.

Government-run disability programs, as humanitarian as their motives are, can be frustrating, with all their red tape and bureaucracy. Workers' Compensation is a prime example. Regardless of what your life was like prior to being injured on the job, there's a good chance that dealing with Worker's Comp will add more stress to it. Just getting your surgery approved can take weeks. Patients often emerge anxious and angry after dealing with the system, and the added stress chemicals can further aggravate pain. By the time they see a surgeon, many Workers' Comp patients have joined the stressed-out B category, with lower chances of a successful outcome. Studies bear this out: Workers' Compensation patients who undergo surgery have less predictable outcomes than non-Workers' Compensation patients (Nguyen).

IA to IB—Stuck in the Disability System

Frank, a productive 30-year-old with good coping skills and a full, rich life (Type IA), ruptured a disc while working onboard a fishing vessel, causing corresponding pain down his leg. This was not Frank's first back injury: he had undergone two decompressions for sciatica five and ten years earlier. By the time he came under my care for the ruptured disc he was frustrated and fed up, having fought the Workers' Comp system for almost a year. He was now in the IB group.

When a patient with an injury like Frank's is facing a third spine operation, it's difficult to know whether to perform another simple decompression or a fusion. We elected to again remove the disc and also performed a fusion. The surgery went well.

During Frank's recovery period over the next six months, he anguished over legal issues and his future occupational prospects. He knew he couldn't go back to being a fisherman, but it was unclear whether Workers' Comp would allow him to train for a new occupation. During his recovery he developed severe anxiety, which evolved into panic attacks. Fortunately, he was under the care of a pain psychologist, and with some medication adjustment he promptly recovered from his anxiety reaction. This additional follow-up support was crucial in helping Frank get through his ordeal. He was finally able to enter a re-training program, and committed to practicing stress management. By addressing all the relevant factors affecting his pain, he was not only able to move on but thrive.

This all happened before I made the connection between chronic pain and anger. Frank easily could have gotten stuck in a pain and disability quagmire. Luckily, with minimal pain and calming down, he entered into the IIA group on his own, which is where he started prior to disc injury. Although he eventually did well, it would have gone so much easier for all of us had he begun the rehab earlier; but I had not yet embraced the prehab approach.

3. Beginning as a IIA (Non-structural Source/ Calm)

Remember Bob, the software engineer with mild scoliosis and sciatica? He had started out in the IA group but became a IB because of complications from an unnecessarily large procedure. Although his problems could have been avoided by limiting his surgery to the only operation he had really needed, at least some procedure was warranted.

The next scenario is even more distressing because there was no identifiable anatomic problem causing pain. Performing surgery on any patient is permanently altering a normal spine. This is a life-changing decision, so both patient and surgeon had better be clear on the justifications—and in the following case there weren't any. A Type IIA patient, formerly enjoying a full and productive existence, will regret this decision for life.

IIA to IB—Normal Spine Fused from Neck to Pelvis

Mike, a forty-year-old steel worker and avid fly fisherman, was struck in the lower back by a steel beam suspended from a cable. Although he was in a lot of pain, he suffered no broken bones, and his spine was normal for his age and active lifestyle. My diagnosis would have been simply a bruised back, which usually subsides with six to twelve weeks of non-operative care. Mike's positive "can-do" attitude qualified him for the A (calm) category.

Instead of non-operative care, though, Mike underwent twelve series of injections in an effort to diagnose the source of his pain based on either stimulating it or relieving it. The test is not reliable enough to diagnose even a structural problem; and, since Mike's pain encompassed his entire spine, this non-specific pattern of pain would be considered non-structural. However, based on the results of these highly subjective tests, he underwent a 12-hour spine fusion from his neck to his pelvis.

When I evaluated Mike about a year after his surgery, he was in constant pain and on high-dose narcotics. He'd gone from being an active outdoorsman to almost completely housebound, unable to walk more than a few blocks without having to sit down. His spine had been fused in a bent-forward position, called "flatback syndrome." He could stand upright only if he bent his knees. Before Mike's injury he was a perennial optimist; but now he was pretty depressed.

In an 11-hour surgery, I realigned Mike's spine and corrected his posture. Within a year he could walk up to two miles and do some fly-fishing. He still required occasional pain medications, but for the most part he was doing well. Since Mike was pretty resilient, his mood improved quickly with minimal intervention. About five years after the surgery, he was doing reasonably well considering what he had been through; but still requiring daily low-dose narcotics for lower back pain.

Although I was able to somewhat salvage Mike's back, his function was not what it would have been without surgical intervention. That unnecessary surgery robbed him of all flexibility from his neck to his pelvis. What helped him as much as my surgery was his inherent optimism and commitment to engaging in his rehab.

As much as was glad I could help Mike live some semblance of a normal life again, I would have much preferred to have gotten to him before his first surgery. Mike is the type that would have done well with simple interventions such as physical therapy, spine education, and vocational counseling. Also, in addition to his needless suffering, he had to bear the costs of two major spine surgeries and two years of intensive medical treatment that included six weeks of physical therapy.

IIA to IB—Partially Paralyzed by an Unnecessary Operation

Rick had recently retired from a career as a middle-school principal when he developed neck pain, a non-structural pain pattern. Even though his MRI scan showed only normal diffuse degeneration for his age, Rick was told he needed surgery. He underwent a fusion through the front of his neck at two levels and a second operation through the back of his neck at four levels. Not only was his neck pain dramatically worse after the surgeries, he woke up after the second operation with both of his shoulders and biceps paralyzed, unable even to raise his hands to feed himself. I worked in conjunction with his pain specialist to help Rick cope with his injury and implemented a comprehensive rehab plan. His neck pain resolved, and he regained a lot of his strength over the next couple of years. But this was not what he had planned for his retirement years.

Retirement is a big change and is often quite stressful for high-energy people like Rick. He hadn't adjusted well to the change. As a IIB Type, he never should have undergone surgery; instead, he would have benefited from minimal engagement in the DOC (Direct your Own Care) process. Now he will spend the rest of his life suffering from complications of unnecessary surgery on his normal, age-appropriate spine.

4. Beginning as a IIB (Non-structural Source/ Hyper-vigilant)

A large percentage of my surgical practice was treating patients who had moved from the IIB category to the IB group. As there had been no identifiable source of pain to begin with, surgery never should have been considered.

Type IIB patients are understandably anxious and frustrated after living with constant pain, earnestly seeking a cure that will bring back their former quality of life, and failing time after time. Therefore, they are the most vulnerable of all the Treatment Grid types when a health professional recommends surgery as an option. Even though no anatomical cause for their pain has been identified, the offer is difficult to refuse, on the off chance that surgery might be the answer.

Surgeons who want to justify a fusion often assign a vague diagnosis called "painful disc," even though there is no inherent reason to perform major surgery just because a disc is "painful." Another unfounded excuse for a fusion is evidence of degeneration on an MRI scan. While it is true that a damaged disc *can* be a source of acute back pain, normal degeneration that occurs with age is not (Boden). It is puzzling—and disturbing—that so many surgeons label age-related degeneration as "abnormal" and use MRI scans to justify thousands of fusions per year in the U.S. (Martin). In response, radiologists have added a standardized paragraph to every spine MRI report pointing out that age-related degenerative disc findings are normal and should not be considered a pain generator (Jarvik).

IIB to IB—Fusions Performed for Nonspecific LBP

Karen, a 43-year-old family housekeeper, while lifting the edge of a mattress one day, felt a "pop" in her back, accompanied by stabbing pain. Neither physical therapy nor four cortisone injections helped; the pain only worsened. During her treatments Karen needed to take off work, and she soon learned her job would not be waiting for her when she recovered.

As a single mother with three children, one of whom had drug-related legal troubles, and no support from her ex-husband, Karen became increasingly sleepless and anxious. Her Workers' Compensation, challenged by her former employer every step of the way, did not cover her bills.

Karen saw several chiropractors and physicians, including a surgeon who ordered an MRI and discograms for the three lowest discs in her back.

A word about discograms: When a disc was thought to be responsible for back pain, surgeons used a test called a discogram to pinpoint which disc was the culprit. The procedure entailed injecting dye into the suspicious disc under x-ray control. Volume and pressure were recorded; and if the patient experienced his or her "usual" back pain while the dye was being injected, it was considered a "positive" result. Interpretation of the test was obviously subjective, making the whole exercise a guessing game. Discograms have since been discredited and are rarely used.

Based on a positive discogram and an MRI that showed normal disc degeneration, Karen's surgeon recommended a fusion of her fourth and fifth vertebrae. The fusion did not relieve her pain. A year later, Karen underwent another fusion, this time on a different level of her spine; but that provided no relief, either. Two years after that, the screws and rods around the fusions were removed with the thought that it might help; but it didn't.

By the time Karen saw me ten years later, I could barely engage with her. She was angry and depressed, and with all the narcotics she was taking could hardly stay awake, Her chronic back pain was now accompanied by severe pain down the front of both legs.

Before her first surgery, Karen was a Type IIB on the Treatment Grid: Her anatomy was non-structural and she was under severe stress. New tests revealed that Karen had a severe constriction of the nerves at L3-4 just above her L4-S1 fusion. With her nerve constriction and anguished mental state, she now belonged in the IB group.

She decided to surgically alleviate her nerve constriction, but we had to wait two months for the state to approve the surgery. Meanwhile, I worked with Karen on her sleep and stress issues. But these problems were so ingrained that her progress was limited. However, I felt Karen's structural problem was compelling enough to first perform the surgery and deal with the rehab issues later.

The surgery consisted of removing the constriction caused by bone and ligaments. We also had to extend her fusion one more level. She was now fused at three levels, but her nerves were no longer constricted. Still, she continued to report pain, as her nervous system had memorized it. Even with my extensive experience with chronic pain, I was astounded; it felt impossible to me that relieving the intense pressure on her nerves wouldn't resolve her leg pain. However, she did reduce her pain medications to a fraction of the pre-op levels, so it seems the surgery had some benefit.

To sum up this sad story: This patient started out in the IIB category. She had no clear structural injury, only some degeneration consistent with her age. However, her condition was complicated by extremely stressful life circumstances. A structured rehabilitation program could have helped, and surgery should not have been considered until after she had engaged in the rehab program. Karen is still in pain and still unable to work.

When the Decision to Have Surgery is Based on Misinformation

Part of your defense against winding up in the IB category is arming yourself with information. Patients sometimes are given justifications for surgery that are simply not true. Here are some of them:

- "If you don't have the surgery you will become paralyzed." Essentially never happens.

- "Back surgery will relieve your back/neck pain." Rarely does spine surgery solve axial pain.

- "You should undergo the operation while you are young and healthy." This is a grey area. Over age 65, there does not seem to be a higher complication rate (Best). However, over age 80, there more medically-related problems related to increased surgical invasion and length of the procedure (Kobayashi).

- "Along with the surgery for your leg (or arm) pain, we're going to add a fusion for your lower back pain." No thanks. Surgery is not effective for LBP, so why "throw it in"? A fusion is a much larger operation than a simple decompression for a pinched nerve.

- "You need a fusion because the surgery might cause instability." Don't buy it. If your surgeon is careful to preserve the facet joints and connecting area of bone (called the *pars*), your spine will not be destabilized. There is less than a 10% chance of destabilization; and if it occurs, your spine can always be fused, then and only then.

- "If you are in a car accident you could be paralyzed." No way. This is a frequent line of reasoning if bone spurs are compressing the spinal cord or nerves, but there are no neurological symptoms. First of all, the chances of complications during surgery are higher than the chances of getting into a motor vehicle accident. And even if an accident should occur, the impact generated by most crashes is too low for such an injury to occur. Rarely, a car accident will cause paralysis regardless of the state of your spine.

If you are fed any of these lines or similar ones, challenge them.

Summary

Beware the IB category. It is particularly tragic if you enter it because of the consequences of spine surgery. You would then be a "failed back surgery syndrome" patient.

If you start out in the IA group, be sure you undergo the simplest operation possible to resolve your pain. An extensive surgery with complications can send you plummeting into the IB category. But if you are already a Type IB (stressed, with a structural source of your pain), you should work on calming down your nervous system to move towards the IA group.

If you are a Type II patient, without a clearly identifiable source of pain, you should not consider spine surgery.

CHAPTER 9

Fusions for Back Pain: A Closer Look

IMAGINE YOU ARE A CONSTRUCTION WORKER who has not missed a day of work in twenty years. One day you injure your lower back on the job. You continue to work, but the minute you mention back pain your employer reproaches you. When you seek medical advice for the pain, your doctor orders you to lay off construction work for a while. You ask your boss for light duty; but your employer refuses to let you return to work until you are back to a 100%. The claims adjuster at your state Workers' Compensation agency fights you every step of the process, suspicious that you are trying to cheat the system.

Meanwhile, none of the treatments prescribed by your doctor help. With no answers or direction, you are finally referred to a surgeon, who diagnoses you with discogenic low back pain. At last: a diagnosis. The surgeon offers you the "definitive treatment: spine fusion," with an implied success rate of 70 - 80%. You desperately want to believe it will work and agree to the procedure. However, it does not work—because you did not have a structural problem treatable by surgery. Now where you can you turn? A major intervention has failed, leaving you with little hope for a solution.

"The Definitive Treatment"

Fusion, the permanent merging of two or more vertebrae, is a major operation with significant complication risks. The classic and appropriate indication for a fusion is that an unstable spine needs to be stabilized. Instability occurs from fractures, tumors, infections and aggressive surgical bone removal.

Yet, one of the most common reasons fusions are performed is to resolve chronic low back pain on an already stable spine, although the chances of relieving LBP with a fusion are low (Martin). Understandably, patients who have exhausted all other options often find surgical intervention difficult to resist, if they feel it offers any chance of relief, no matter how small.

In this chapter we will draw upon research findings that demonstrate why fusions are *not* a viable treatment for non-specific lower back pain. We'll explore the evidence by Treatment Grid patient groups, in the following order:

- Fusions for Types IA and IIA— If the disc really is the source of pain and their nervous systems are calm, these patients should do well with surgery.

- Fusions for Type IIB—Outcomes are predictably poor for patients with no identifiable sources of pain and fired-up nervous systems.

- Fusions vs. structured, non-operative care: No advantages of surgery over organized non-operative care for chronic LBP.

- The sole paper used to justify fusions for LBP: Rife with flaws.

But before delving into the studies that invalidate the practice of performing fusions for LBP, following is a brief outline of the arguments and supporting evidence.

The Case Against Surgery for Chronic Low Back Pain: An Overview

In general, fusions for LBP are erroneously justified by diagnoses of "degenerative disc disease" and "discogenic back pain."

- Degenerative changes of the discs are *not* sources of chronic LBP. This includes bulging, ruptured, or herniated discs; bone spurs, arthritis or stable malalignment of the vertebra (spondylolisthesis) (Jarvik, Boden). Many radiology reports now include the statement that such findings are considered normal age-related changes. The only exception occurs when degeneration erodes the facet joints enough to allow excessive motion and create instability; but this happens only occasionally. In general, faulty or diseased discs do not cause chronic low back pain.

- Degeneration usually creates *more* stability, because the reduction in water content causes the disc to become stiffer, allowing less motion. When the disc finally collapses and becomes "bone on bone," it essentially has almost fused on its own, becoming even more stable, and therefore less likely a source of pain. The facets at the back of the spine also expand, adding even more support.

- Even if a disc was the source of pain, we have no test to accurately diagnose which disc. The pertinent research papers do not clarify how the surgeons decided which levels to fuse (Fritzell, Carragee).

- When acute pain becomes chronic, associated brain activity moves from the acute pain area to the emotional area of the brain, where it is memorized (Hashmi). Structural intervention cannot possibly work for neurological issues.

- No study supports back fusion as a better treatment for back pain than even mildly structured non-operative care (Fritzell, Brox, Fairbanks).

- The success rate for a lumbar fusion in the best studies is less then 30% at a two-year follow up (Carragee). The few studies that show a higher success rate (>70%) were performed in centers that provided a strong structured rehab program (Brox, Fairbanks).

- Significant complications and re-operation rates occur within two years of surgery (Kerezoudis).

- Only 10% of spine surgeons are addressing the risk factors for poor outcomes before proceeding with surgery (Young).

- Operating on patients with untreated chronic pain can induce or worsen the pain up to 40 - 50% of the time, up to a year; the pain becomes permanent 5 - 10% of the time (Perkins, Schug).

An alternative to fusion is replacing a degenerated disc with an artificial one. This procedure allows for motion, theoretically lessening the risk of future breakdown around a fusion. But the fact still remains that the disc is not a proven source of low back pain; so the procedure is likely to be an ineffective and unnecessary risk.

Results of Fusions for LBP in Types IA and IIA Patients

Let's first look at the outcomes of fusions for Type A patients. Remember that these patients are coping relatively well with their chronic lower back pain. But whereas the IA patient has an identifiable source of pain clearly visible on an imaging test, the IIA patient has no identifiable source of pain. If a Type IIA patient agreed to surgery, what would be the chances of a successful outcome? This question has been examined in one of the most carefully executed studies in spine research (Carragee).

Dr. Eugene Carragee at Stanford University compared lumbar fusions performed on two groups of patients: One group had a visible structural instability (Type I), and the other group had presumed "discogenic pain" (Type II). His hypothesis was that, if the discogram was a valid test to accurately diagnose one or more discs to be the source of pain, then a fusion that removes the structural problem should solve patients' back pain.

The principle behind a discogram is that, if a disc is pressurized with dye injected directly into it, and the pressure replicates the patient's "usual back pain," then the disc must be the source of pain. Dr. Carragee challenged the idea that "discogenic pain" based on a positive discogram was a valid diagnosis, by taking extremely precise measurements of the volume of fluid, the pressure created within the disc, and the patients' reported pain.

In the discogenic group, he performed fusions only if a carefully scrutinized discography revealed the presence of a damaged or abnormal disc at L4-5 or L5-S1. Patients' stress profiles were also reviewed, and only those patients with few psychosocial risk factors (Type A) for chronic pain were included. Back pain is a vague, nonspecific symptom (Type II); and the discogram has not been shown to be a valid test for localizing source of pain. Therefore, in our terms, this "discogenic group" is in the Type IIA quadrant of the Treatment Grid.

Patients with an identifiable source of pain (Type I) had a distinct structural problem. Lamina in the back of their spines had a bony defect on each side and weren't attached to the front (isthmic spondylolisthesis). Dr. Carragee chose only patients who had over four millimeters of movement when bending backwards and forwards. This is considered quite unstable and a structural problem. The patients in this group were also carefully screened for low stress with validated questionnaires. Therefore, they were Type IA: identifiable pain source and calm.

The results showed that the "discogenic," IIA group had a surgical success rate of only 27% as compared to 72% for the structural, IA group. Success was defined by the patients' satisfaction with the degree of pain relief two years after the fusion.

This study was surprising to me for two reasons. First, I thought the success rate for the unstable spondylolisthesis would be higher than 72%. The results reinforced my opinion that, even in the face of an identifiable source of low back pain, the soft tissues around the spine should be treated first. There is always the chance that the pain will diminish enough that surgery can be avoided.

Second, I was surprised that the success rate for the discogenic group was so low (27%), especially given the fact that all the patients were in the calm category. Even with my bias toward noninvasive treatment, the surgeon in me still believes that, if I could pinpoint a problem disc with a high-quality discography, I could perform a successful fusion in this carefully selected patient group. But that expectation was not borne out by the study. Imagine if the discography group had a IIB profile, with a hyper-vigilant rather than calm nervous system. It is unlikely that even 27% would have benefited from the fusion.

Proponents of fusions might argue that the size of the study was too small to be definitive, with only thirty patients in each group. However, as carefully controlled as it was over five years, its quality is unmatched in the field. I believe it is to date the most important paper to examine the effectiveness of fusions for LBP.

I used discograms as the basis for performing fusions for back pain during my early years of practice. In retrospect, I see major flaws with this test.

- Patients' pain experience varies from day to day. How can you characterize your "usual" pain? This measurement is highly subjective and vague.

- The radiologist or surgeon interprets the patient's report of pain. This leaves room for more subjectivity and variability.

- If too much dye is injected into any disc too quickly—even a healthy one—it will cause pain. The technique of measuring pressure, volume and speed of the dye infusion contain significant variability.

It isn't reasonable to perform a major surgical intervention based on such an unreliable test. In spite of Dr. Carragee demonstrating its unreliability, discograms are still widely used as the basis for a lumbar fusion.

Results of Fusions for LBP in IIB Patients (Non-structural/Hyper-vigilant)

Now let's explore chronic pain treatment for those who are not coping well with their pain. Perhaps they are anxious about treatment outcomes; perhaps they under a lot of stress because of life crises unrelated to their pain. If this is you, you are a Type B, and your nervous system is fired up. Under these circumstances it is difficult to sustain relief from surgical intervention alone.

Imagine you've been told the source of your pain is a degenerated disc (Type II, since degenerated discs are not reliable sources of LBP), and that surgery is the definitive treatment for your condition. What are your chances of being satisfied with a fusion or disc replacement? One answer comes from Gary Franklin, MD, and medical director of Worker's Compensation in the state of Washington. Dr. Franklin examined the outcomes of spine fusions for lower back pain in injured workers (Franklin).

As I've described earlier in the book, the journey through the Workers' Comp system is enough to push most patients into the B group. Between the injury, unsympathetic case administrators, resistant employers and bureaucratic delays, it's an uphill struggle. Dr. Franklin studied 388 patients who had undergone fusions for low back problems between 1986 and 1987. Each patient had back pain, leg pain, or both, with a mixture of degenerative diagnoses. Instability was not documented, so there may have been some structural patients included.

Analysis of two-year follow up data revealed a return-to-work rate average of 16% at one year, 32% at two years, and 49% at the three-year follow-up. At every time interval, the return-to-work was less than that of a comparable group of patients who had not undergone a fusion.

Sixty-five percent of the patients responded to a follow up questionnaire. Of the responders, 68% said the pain was the same or worse than before the operation. Factors that predicted a poorer outcome were older age, longer time on disability before having surgery, a greater number of levels fused, and a higher number of prior low back surgeries.

This study has been criticized for several reasons, including the fact that it was not a controlled, randomized study (wherein similar patients are randomly placed into different treatment groups and then compared). The study also had only a 65% follow-up rate at two years from the surgery. There was also a mixture of diagnoses.

I agree with these criticisms, but I still think the study is a valid snapshot of how patients with lumbar fusions will fare. I also believe the criticisms highlight the fact that, thirty years later, the medical profession still hasn't come up with another study to validate fusions in this population. The data is more negative of performing fusions for LBP, and the burden of proof validating this operation is in the medical profession's court.

In 2006, a similar study of Washington Workers' Compensation patients looked at 1,950 fusion operations performed between 1994 and 2001, in which the primary indication was low back pain (Sham). The study drew from database records, so statistics were available for 100% of the patients. This time the surgeons used spinal cages— hollow cylinders or rectangles that are filled with bone graft and placed between vertebral bodies after removing disc material. With the increased support and graft provided by the cages, there is a higher chance of obtaining a solid fusion.

The overall disability rate two years after the fusion was 64%, with a 22% re-operation rate. Since these patients were treated with advanced technology (the spinal cages), theoretically the patients should have exhibited improved outcomes. But no difference was found between patients who had received spinal cages and those who did not.

While I was practicing medicine in Idaho from 1998 to 2003, I spoke to many Workers' Comp claims examiners who regularly dealt with injured workers before and after surgery for non-specific back pain. These conversations came about as a result of my trying to put together a network of surgeons who were willing to institute a defined program of non-operative care to treat non-specific low back pain, with the idea that it would be required for patients looking to undergo a lumbar fusion. I found that the claims examiners not only felt that the surgery was ineffective; they could recall very few cases where it had ever worked.

When I first began performing fusions for LBP in 1986, Seattle and the surrounding communities were enthusiastically performing these back pain fusions. We had been introduced to new technology in the form of pedicle screws, which enhanced our ability to create a solid fusion. There wasn't much data and we assumed the new procedure would be effective. I spent almost eight years performing this operation before Dr. Franklin's paper was published. I immediately stopped performing fusions for disc degeneration in any patient with LBP.

I'd estimate most patients expect an 80 - 90% success rate from a fusion for LBP. When I told my patients that the success rate is less than 30%, they usually lost their interest in surgery (Carragee, Franklin).

Results of Fusions for Low Back Pain versus Structured Non-operative Care

Brox's Study

Brox compared results from surgery to results from carefully structured, non-operative care in 64 patients between the ages of 25 and 60. His anatomic criterion was merely disc degeneration noted on x-rays, with more than one year of persistent back pain. He did not report what tests he used to identify the exact level of degeneration.

Other criteria were used to exclude patients from the study, most notably stress. Hence, patients were in the IIA group (no identifiable pain source/calm). One would expect that both the surgical and non-surgical patients would respond reasonably well to almost any treatment.

The surgical group (those receiving fusions) consisted of 37 patients and the non-surgical, 27. Fusions were performed only from the back, with 84% of the fusions becoming solid. The non-operative treatment consisted of twenty-five hours of body mechanics, education, and cognitive behavioral therapy focused on improving compliance with physical therapy. They had one week of intensive treatment, one week off at home, and then finished with an intensive two-week session.

The success rate of the surgical group was 71%, with an early complication rate of 18%. The success rate of the non-surgical group was 76%. It was concluded that surgery did not offer any benefit over structured, non-operative care. (And even if the non-operative group's success rate had been slightly less, it must be noted that rehab avoids the complication risk associated with a fusion.)

I was initially surprised at the high rate of success for the surgical group. A rate of 71% is much higher than most surgical series. However, one must take into account that all patients were IIA; careful psychological testing had screened out anyone who was under heavy stress. It also explains why the non-operative care worked so well: Type IIA patients are better able to engage in a fairly aggressive, complex rehab regimen. It's likely that some of the same health providers were treating both groups, so I suspect that the rehab in the surgical group was better than the usual rehab—another reason why they would have done well.

Overall, the biggest problem I saw with this study was that, once the funding for the study ran out, it seemed the structured non-operative resources disappeared. Dr. Brox's final comment in the paper was that "structured, non-operative care was not widely available." This means that the patients who had done well with rehab would no longer have access to those resources, putting them at risk for a relapse. What about those who could potentially avoid surgery? If a fraction of the money spent on fusions were used to develop and sustain a structured care program, the benefits would greatly outweigh the costs.

Fairbanks's Study

Dr. Fairbanks published the results of a large study based in England that randomly divided back pain patients between fusion and rigorous non-operative care. The surgeons decided which levels were to be fused, and the criteria they used were not specified. If imaging was used in the decision-making process, it wasn't noted; hence, the surgery appeared to be somewhat of a random event. The non-operative care consisted of general exercise programs for muscle strengthening, flexibility training, cardiovascular endurance and cognitive behavioral therapy.

There was a slight advantage of surgery over non-operative care, but the difference was minimal. No apparent benefit of surgery was found over structured rehab, especially considering the risks and costs of surgery. Overall, 75% of people were able to avoid surgery with this level of rehab. The final conclusion was similar to the Brox study in that a comprehensive rehab approach wasn't widely available, although it should have been. Obstacles cited were finances, space and training. But that is a strongly debatable point, because the costs of surgery are great, especially when they fail. In this case, 11 of 176 surgical patients returned to the OR for a complication.

The Sole Paper Used to Justify Fusions for Back Pain

A solid research study is characterized by subjects randomly assigned to experimental and control groups, with neither the subjects (patients) nor the researchers (doctors) knowing which subjects are assigned to each group. Results are analyzed while controlling for as many variables as possible (characteristics that could influence the outcome), such as age and medical history; and involve enough subjects to reasonably form a conclusion—the more the better.

There are no solid research papers that compare the effectiveness of a fusion for LBP with well-defined non-operative care. The following paper is the most cited study in support of fusions, although the data is weak. While the patients were randomly assigned to the four treatments, they had the final say whether they would undergo surgery.

Dr. Fritzell's Study

One of Fritzell's papers, published in 2004, is considered a landmark study in support of fusions for low back pain. In it, Dr. Fritzell compared surgery to what he called "the usual conservative care." However, I believe his conclusions were based on a flawed research design, beginning with the fact that the non-operative care consisted of doing nothing different from that which had already failed to solve the back pain. A better description would have been "non-care." In addition, a spinal implant manufacturer funded the study, so the element of bias cannot be ruled out.

The surgical group had 222 patients and the non-surgical group 72. The three-to-one ratio of surgical to non-surgical patients resulted from the fact that they were comparing three different hardware constructs to obtain a solid fusion. There was no effort made to see if surgery should be performed or what might be the most effective way to avoid surgery. It is one of the chief reasons why this paper should not be used to justify the effectiveness of a fusion for pain.

The non-surgical group received various treatments but there was no structure in place to determine the level of care received or what treatments were used. Essentially, it was the same "non-care" that had already failed. As the patients had each been in pain for around eight years, one wouldn't expect much improvement. Indeed, in the end, there was very little improvement observed.

In the surgical group, a lumbar fusion was performed for degenerative disc disease on one or both of the two lowest levels of the spine at L4-5 and L5-S1. These are Type II patients because LBP is non-specific and there are not any reliable diagnostic tests to pinpoint the pain source. The surgical decision was based two findings: 1) X-rays showing degeneration; and 2) patients' reports of pain when the doctor applied direct pressure to the lower back, without x-ray confirmation of the level receiving the pressure.

This selection criteria for surgery negates all findings of the study. First of all, pushing on someone's back while lying prone is not a valid test to determine which, if any, disc is the source of pain. Pain can arise from any of the layers of tissue (fascia) enveloping muscles. The ligaments holding the spine together also contain many pain receptors. Even if the disc was causing pain, how do we know that pushing on the skin would confirm it? There is a much higher chance that a spot that is tender to the touch is the result of soft tissues around the spine, rather than the spinal column itself.

A classic example is fibromyalgia, where many areas throughout the body—including the low back—are tender to the touch. In this study, fibromyalgia was overlooked as a possible diagnosis. What is equally disturbing was that, even if pushing on the skin was a valid test, how did the surgeon know where he or she was pushing? The only reliable way is to take an x-ray while pressure is being applied. Otherwise it is impossible to know the exact level, especially in large patients. Incidentally, operating at the wrong level of the spine is the most common error in spine surgery even with x-ray control. One could easily conclude that Fritzell et al. performed random fusions.

Another glitch was that this study factored in the presence of bone spurs as a possible source of LBP, even though the literature has failed to identify any connection to LBP (Boden).

One key variable that was not clearly documented was the patients' levels of stress. Those with "obvious psychiatric illness" were excluded; but the number of patients with sensitized nervous systems was not known. The length of pain and disability suffered by the patients in the study make it likely that most, if not all, patients were in the hyper-vigilant, Type B group; and this fact could have influenced the results in both groups.

Even though this was a well-funded, relatively large study, the diagnostic criteria were invalid and the non-operative care in the non-surgical group was neither defined nor monitored. Given the weak premises on which the study rested, the results of the study are questionable.

The surgical group had a fairly impressive decrease in pain during a six-month, post-surgical period. However, at two-year follow-up the pain had significantly increased, and the final average improvement in pain was only about 30%. The improvement in function was 25%. Depression decreased about 20%.

The non-surgical group had an average improvement in pain of 7%, improved function of 6%, and decrease in depression of 7%. Since the surgical group had a "statistically better improvement" than the non-operative (non-care) group, the conclusion was that a lumber fusion was a valid intervention for back pain. Remember, the focus of the study was to determine the best of three methods to obtain a solid fusion, not to compare surgery with non-operative care.

The patients in the surgical group did have statistically greater improvement (better than chance) than the non-surgical group in pain, function and depression, although the overall outcomes were dismal. But it's clear that the non-surgical group had essentially no structured non-operative treatment such as addressing social isolation, sleep, stress, medication, physical conditioning, or family dynamics. In fact, I am surprised that there was any improvement at all in the non-surgical group, because untreated chronic pain usually worsens over time, even without additional injury (Gieseke).

In a commentary on Fritzell's study, prominent spine surgeon Vert Mooney wrote that the non-surgical group's care was the equivalent of non-care (Mooney). He was concerned that this paper would be used as the basis for justifying the ongoing use of spine surgery as a treatment for low back pain. It appears that Dr. Mooney's concerns were founded.

Now let's look at the complications Dr. Fritzell's patients experienced. The overall complication rate was 24% (50 of 211 surgeries), with 8% (16 of 211) requiring additional, unplanned surgeries. The complications included three nerves hit by a screw (requiring reoperation); two non-healing fusions (reoperation); five deep wound infections; one patient operated on at the wrong level; and six introductions of new nerve root pain. There were also seven patients who experienced potentially life-threatening complications, including two major bleeds during the abdominal approach, two blood clots in the legs (with one resulting in the clot traveling to the lungs [pulmonary embolus]), one case of pneumonia, one fluid overload of the lungs, and one heart failure with bleeding from the gastrointestinal tract.

Other complications requiring additional surgery included: two hematomas (excessive bleeding) at the donor site for the bone graft from the pelvis; two superficial skin problems; and one patient with damage to the sensory nerve running down the front of his leg. Other complications not requiring more surgery included three gastrointestinal bleeds, two screws placed outside the spinal canal, two cases of damage to the sympathetic nerves with observed symptoms (usually a temperature difference between legs or abnormal tingling sensations), one dural tear (leakage of spinal fluid), one case of unexplained arm pain, nine cases of pain at the bone graft site, and one instance of abnormal motion of the shoulder blade.

Other Marginal Indications for Spine Surgery

In this chapter I focused on one procedure—lumbar fusion for chronic low back pain—to underscore its senselessness. I chose this particular operation because it is the most commonly performed unnecessary surgery. However, there are several other equally non-indicated spinal surgeries worthy of mention:

- Cervical fusions for neck pain

- Long fusions for balanced spinal deformity (There is minimal evidence that either scoliosis or kyphosis is a source of pain.)

- Laminectomies and discectomies for back pain

- Sacral iliac joint fusions for SI joint pain

- Fusions for fractures that could be stabilized with a brace

- Decompressions for pinched nerves, when there is enough fluid around the nerves to rule out nerve compression

- Surgery based on miscommunication between patient and surgeon (For example, the patient thinks the surgery will address axial pain while the surgeon is treating radicular pain.)

- Surgery performed before considering and addressing all factors that influence pain perception

Summary

There is no compelling evidence to support fusion as a viable option for chronic low back pain. In fact, fifty years from now, we'll probably be looking back at this era of out-of-control spine surgery the way we now view our craze for frontal lobotomies in the mid-1900s. It took several decades to discredit and abandon that procedure. Lumbar fusion for LBP isn't an overused operation; it shouldn't be used at all.

In considering fusions, we must ask, do they ever work for axial back pain? The answer is yes, sometimes, for a structural, unstable vertebral motion segment (vertebra-disc-vertebra); and the results can be dramatic. But a success rate under 30% on stable, degenerated spines is unacceptable (Carragee, Franklin, Nguyen)— especially when studies have failed to find it better than structured non-operative care. The problem with a spine fusion is that there is always a downside. Your spine is stiffer, the pain may become worse, your spine can develop a severe deformity, stenosis, or fractures around the ends of the fusion, and the list goes on.

It is difficult to put into words the horror stories and disasters I have witnessed. Here's where it starts: If you have a failed surgery— or, more likely, multiple failed surgeries—you have permanent structural damage to your spine, in addition to the chronic pain that brought you to surgery in the first place.

Once your condition is labeled "failed back syndrome," you will find it even more difficult to find doctors who will accept you as a patient. Many physicians are reluctant to take on someone else's failures. In addition, few surgeons are trained in dealing with chronic pain.

In surgeons' defense, we want to help our patients and we want good outcomes. There is a high demand for fusions because patients in pain desperately want to find a way out of their misery. Since we surgeons feel that we are the "last resort," we want to meet our patients' needs.

At the same time, our current healthcare system severely limits the time we can spend with our patients, so we are working with limited information about them. Interventions that reduce chronic pain without surgery are not consistently covered by insurance. Hospitals monitor doctors for their "contribution to the profit margin," based on delivering services that are profitable regardless of their effectiveness. While this practice is true in every field of medicine, it is particularly treacherous for spine patients because of the enormous downside to a failed spine operation.

SECTION 4:
LEARN THE DETAILS

Know Your Diagnosis

WE HAVE DISCUSSED THE OVERALL concepts that determine whether an anatomical finding is a structural (Type I) or a non-structural problem (Type II). Adding to these straightforward criteria, there is one more wrinkle: Of the various diagnoses we use to define abnormalities of the spine, each has its own unique characteristics, which determine which group they belong in. This section will explore those differences and allow you to answer the question: "Is my *particular diagnosis* structural or non-structural?" Or, said a different way, "Is my *particular diagnosis* amenable to surgery or not?"

We define elective surgery as that performed at the patient's request because of pain or deformity. Non-elective surgery is performed for problems that are damaging, destructive, or progressive, which only surgery has a chance of solving. The most common diagnoses treated with elective spine surgery are:

1. Degenerative disc disease

2. Ruptured or herniated discs

3. Spinal stenosis

4. Spondylolisthesis

    – Degenerative

    – Isthmic

5. Spinal deformity

   – Scoliosis

   – Kyphosis

6. Compression fractures

To make a final determination whether your problem is amenable to surgery, review the concepts in Chapter 3 that define structural and non-structural sources of symptoms. Then look up your specific diagnosis from the above list and apply those concepts to your specific situation.

The following patterns of pain were presented in chapter 3:

- Axial

- Radicular

- Claudication

If the problem is a neurological deficit instead of or in addition to pain, it is considered a spine structural problem as long as there is a corresponding anatomical lesion in the spinal column—although lesions occurring elsewhere in the body can cause neurological compromise as well. In the event of impending or progressive neurological deficits, decisions need to be made quickly and definitively. Your medical team will be very clear about this when they discuss your condition with you. Not all such scenarios are treated surgically; but if they were, it would not be a case of elective surgery, which is most often based on your level of pain. This book is intended to help you make a good decision about *elective* surgery, so it isn't focused on neurological issues.

1. Degenerative Disc Disease

Disc degeneration is normal as we age and *not* a source of ongoing pain (Boden). A more accurate term for degenerative disc disease is "normally aging discs." If you have only neck, thoracic or low back pain (axial pain) and you've been told that you have degenerative disc disease, you are in the Type II, non-structural section of the grid. Axial pain is just too diffuse and non-specific to be classified as structural. In this case, surgery is not indicated.

Of course, the presence of "red flag" symptoms indicates potential serious problems (Chapter 3); but disc degeneration in itself is still not the cause of pain. Another source of pain might be a partial tear of the rings of the disc, called an *annular tear* (discussed later in this section), which can bring on acute, sudden pain. However, although this is an anatomical injury, it is still considered non-structural, because the symptoms are vague and widespread, and testing can't determine which disc the pain is coming from. You may also have been told that you have the following problems causing your axial pain:

- Bone spurs

- Arthritis

- Bulging, herniated, or ruptured discs

- Facet pain

- Bone-on-bone or collapsed discs

As daunting as these diagnoses sound, none has been proven to cause axial pain in any area of the spine. In truth, we know the source of axial pain only 5 - 15% of the time (Nachemson). Said another way, if you decide on surgery for axial pain, the surgeon is guessing where the problem is over 85% of the time.

Disc Anatomy and Function

Each vertebra is separated by a structure called an *intervertebral disc*. The disc provides several functions:

- Allowing motion between the vertebrae

- Acting as a spacer, which allows the nerves to exit at the disc level from the central spinal canal

- Providing protective feedback including position and pain sensation

The center of the disc, the *nucleus*, is made of semi-gelatinous material with a high water content but no blood supply or nerve fibers. The nucleus is encircled by a ring called the *annulus*, whose many layers are arranged at a 60-degree angle to the nucleus, each layer oriented opposite the one before, similar to the plies of a radial tire. The annulus has a rich nerve supply that transmits pain (*nociception*) and tells your brain where you are in space (*proprioception*). Small tears in the annulus (*annular tears*) may be one reason for acute lower back pain, by allowing the nuclear material to come in contact with the pain receptors in the ring. However, this condition usually resolves quickly and is not a reason to perform surgery.

The disc works most efficiently when direct compression is exerted across it, which occurs while a person is in the upright position. As force is vertically applied to the nucleus, horizontal hydraulic forces are generated, which pushes against the annulus. The load is also shared by two facet joints on each disc, which are locked in place at the back of the spinal column.

The disc's construct is similar to that of a three-legged stool. It is extremely strong and stable, with the cushion in front stabilized by the two facet joints in the back. If you are lifting a heavy object properly—from an upright position, taking most of the weight in your legs—the semi-liquid central hydraulic effect becomes stronger with more direct compression.

But if you lift something heavy from a bent-over posture, the opposite effect occurs. The facet joints unlock and cannot share the load. Instead of a strong hydraulic effect on the disc, the forces are now shearing across it and tearing it down. Additionally, there is a lever-arm effect that magnifies the forces based on the distance the force is applied from the center of the disc.

Over time the discs will gradually wear down; and, combined with losing water content as we age, will degenerate. A worn disc cannot regenerate itself. Even though this process happens to all of us, several factors can affect the rate at which it occurs. Some factors are:

- Amount of repetitive bending
- Genetics
- Physical condition of the body (your "core" strength; aerobic activity)
- Smoking

As the water content of the disc decreases, there is less of a hydraulic effect, and more force is exerted on the annulus (the ring around the nucleus) and facet joints. There is now more pressure on the perimeter of vertebral body, causing the formation of bone spurs. These are not a problem as long as nerves are not pinched. Less water content also causes the nucleus to shrink and the ring to gradually break down. The space between the vertebra narrows and the spine becomes less flexible. The vertebrae may almost touch each other or become "bone on bone," essentially fusing themselves. Although this whole process sounds perilous, it's not. It is descriptive of normal aging and therefore not considered a structural source of pain.

As the disc shrinks, the facet joints in the back of the spine are also affected, altering the normal relationship between the opposing surfaces and causing the normal cartilage to break down, resulting in arthritis. Whether facet arthritis is a cause of low back pain is a hotly debated topic.

Additionally, the space for the exiting nerves is decreased as the disc settles, which can compress the nerves. The pressure can cause weakness, numbness, and/or pain down the distribution of the nerve.

In a nutshell, discs normally lose water and become stiffer with age. Since water provides the signals that register in MRI scans, less hydration produces a darker disc on a scan. That's all there is to it; the darker areas do not indicate pathologic anatomy that causes pain. It's not a state of disease; it's a normally occurring process.

Normally aging spines also lose their youthful flexibility, but a less flexible spine doesn't mean a painful spine. Several studies of the cervical, thoracic, and lumbar spine have demonstrated that there is little correlation between a degenerated, herniated, bulging, or ruptured disc and axial pain (Boden, Jarvik). For example, if you randomly study one hundred people who have **never** experienced significant low back pain, by age fifty over half will have bone spurs, arthritis, herniated or ruptured discs, disc bulges, and/or "degenerative disc disease." By age sixty-five, the number approaches 100% of the pain-free group. In an effort to increase awareness that these are normal, age-related findings, radiologists now document that these findings are a part of the normal aging process and clinical correlation is recommended.

Severe Degeneration and No LBP

I evaluated a fifty-year-old woman who was experiencing sharp pain down the side of her left leg when she stood up and walked. She was an avid cyclist, runner, and regular at the gym. Her imaging study revealed narrowing around her fifth lumbar nerve root as it exited her spine. Every time she stood up it tightly pinched the nerve. In addition, her spine was one of the worst looking spines I have ever seen. Every disc was completely collapsed, each vertebra was "bone against bone," and there was a moderate amount of curvature. But this patient had absolutely no back pain, and there had been none in her past. I performed a one-level fusion at L5-S1, which prevented the opening around her 5th nerve from collapsing when she stood up and relieved the pressure on the nerve. Her leg pain was gone, she never developed back pain, and she went back to full activities, with her "terrible-looking" spine.

Chronic Axial Pain with Disc Degeneration is Non-structural

What makes this case so interesting is that surgeons see patients every day with "terrible-looking spines" and no back or neck pain. Usually the patient is there for a pinched nerve that is causing leg or arm pain. But if a patient comes in with only neck or back pain, suddenly the degeneration "must be the source" of pain. It is completely illogical, especially when the same reasoning is used for performing major surgery. Most of the discs in almost everyone's lower back have some degeneration. Even if you thought one of them might be a source of pain, how do you know which one it is? There is no diagnostic test accurate enough to identify it. Even the more invasive testing procedure of injecting dye into the disc has been found to be unreliable and is no longer widely done (Carragee).

This is not to say that discs can never be the source of pain. They *can* cause pain in the initial acute phase of an injury, but usually the disc is reasonably hydrated, with more movement than a partially narrowed, degenerated disc. The ring around the perimeter of the disc can be torn, irritating the nerve fibers in the disc, which can be quite painful. However, it is a different pain pattern than that of chronic low back pain.

Even Acute Discogenic Pain is Non-structural

As we discussed above, disc degeneration is part of the normal aging process and should not be blamed for chronic lower back pain. There are times, however, when it can be a source of a *different kind of pain*, other than chronic LBP.

Discogenic pain—the term given to back pain caused by one or more discs—is usually episodic and severe. Often there are intense muscle spasms and an "involuntary shift" of the upper body over the pelvis. Usually there is no pain between the episodes, which last a few days to several weeks. Since sitting increases internal disc pressure, most physicians believe that if the pain is worse while sitting, then the disc is to blame (Nachemson). The overall pattern is that the pain eventually calms down with good non-operative care; or the disc may rupture, at which time the (axial) LBP is replaced by radicular pain. Excellent posture, body mechanics and physical conditioning are critical for patients addressing discogenic pain. But the pain pattern is vague and we have no test to localize which disc might be the source; therefore it is still a non-structural problem.

But the pain pattern that most often drives a patient to undergo surgery is the *opposite* of what I just described as discogenic pain. Daily, constant pain that lasts for months or years is more likely to stem from strains, sprains or inflammation of the muscles, tendons, fascial layers, or ligaments around the spine. Almost any activity aggravates it. Embedded pain circuits can remain active after the acute injury has healed, requiring an approach that calms the nervous system in order to resolve (Hashmi). Also, the brain can spontaneously generate severe pain in any part of the body. We don't completely understand why this can happen, but it may be related to the body's chemistry, which changes the pain threshold. The brain also may simply "short circuit." Chapter 6 explains this in more detail.

This section is intended to give you a feel that *one very definite cause of low back pain* can be the disc. The pattern, I feel, is severe, episodic, with the intervals being pain free. Nonetheless, this situation still does not fit my proposed definition of an identifiable pain source. It must be accurately identified on a diagnostic test and have matching symptoms. There is no test that will identify which disc the pain is originating from. *After* the disc ruptures, I think it is reasonable to assume that the low back pain originated from the disc that ruptured—especially if the LBP disappears. But before a rupture we simply don't have accurate enough diagnostic tools to figure it out.

2. Ruptured or Herniated Disc

A ruptured disc, also known as a herniated disc, occurs when the disc's central nuclear material pushes through all of the layers of rings of the annulus. It can occur in any direction but is usually a problem only when it enters the spinal canal. As the rings give way, the annulus starts to buckle before it breaks, similar to a bubble that occurs in the weak part of an inner tube. The descriptive term at this stage is a "bulging disc". When the nuclear material is in the canal, a thin layer of tissue may contain it, or it may break free (a "free fragment"). The disc may rupture and compress nerves without causing any pain, weakness, or numbness down the leg.

When pain or neurological symptoms appear down the arm or leg along the pathway of a specific nerve, the medical term is *radicular pain*. The locations of pain associated with the different lumbar nerves are:

- **First sacral (S1)**—Back of the upper leg, back of the calf, side and/or bottom of the foot
- **Fifth lumbar (L5)**—Side of the upper leg, side of the calf, top of the foot, big toe
- **Fourth lumbar (L4)**—Front of the upper leg, front of the lower leg (shin)
- **Third lumbar (L3)**—Groin and kneecap
- **Second lumbar (L2)**—Groin and inside of thigh

KNOW YOUR DIAGNOSIS | 141

The pain can be in just part of the distribution of the nerve. For example, the 6th cervical nerve travels down the side of the shoulder, outside the upper arm and forearm and to the thumb. The pain from an irritated or pinched 6th cervical nerve may be located only in the shoulder or thumb. Or it may travel down the whole length of the nerve. In the lower back the 5th lumbar nerve travels down the buttock, side of the thigh and calf, top of the foot and into the big toe. The pain can be located in just the big toe or in the buttocks. Localized pain seems to occur more often than pain down the whole nerve.

The onset of pain is usually rapid over several hours, although it might build up gradually with back pain and spasms over several days or weeks. Usually the pain is severe for a few days, but then it calms down within a couple of weeks. If the pain is going to abate without surgery, you'll usually experience some improvement within eight to twelve weeks.

A key element of a disc rupture is that the material pushing on the nerve root is usually soft. There is potential for the body to reabsorb it and for the extruded nuclear material to shrink or even disappear with resolution of the radicular pain. We weren't aware of this process until the introduction of MRI scans in the 1980's, when it became safe to restudy patients without additional radiation exposure. Several studies showed that large disc ruptures in the neck or lower back could reabsorb within a year of the original event (Ribeiro, Shan). Initially, I had a certain level of disbelief that this was possible, but I witnessed it several times during my career. A patient would come in with a classic ruptured disc and radicular pain. We were able to resolve the pain non-operatively with medications, epidural steroid injections, and time. Maybe a year of two later the same pain would return to the point where I felt it necessary to rescan the area. The ruptured disc was gone. It had disappeared. I now understand that the recurrent pain was from the triggering of prior memorized neurological circuits. That pain would cease over several weeks using an approach that included addressing the nervous system component.

Occasionally, part of the bony section of the disc, the end plate, will rupture; these don't reabsorb. The ring around the disc (annulus) is also firm. A diagnostic test such as an MRI does not reveal whether the rupture is hard or soft material. A soft rupture will begin to resolve fairly quickly, while the end plate or annular rupture won't improve and often worsens. The only way you can assess it is to follow it over time, and the definitive determination of the type of material can be made only during surgery.

Miscellaneous Factors

A disc rupture can occur in four different spots at any level of the spine.

- The middle of the spinal canal: There is generally plenty of room for the nerves, and even very large ruptures may not cause any leg pain or weakness.

- To one side of the spinal canal: This is the most common location for a disc rupture. It can trap the nerve just before it exits the side of the spinal canal. Most disc ruptures occur at the two lowest levels, L4-5 and L5-S1 or in the middle of the cervical spine between the 4th and 5th or 5th and 6th vertebra.

- In the foramen: If the disc rupture occurs within one of the small holes on the side of the spinal canal (foramina), the pain is frequently intense, and may have a lower chance of improving *without* surgery.

- The far lateral area (*extraforaminal*): Once it has exited the foramina, the nerve has more room; but the disc rupture can still be large enough to trap the nerve and cause a lot of pain. Such a "far lateral" disc rupture is treacherous for a couple of reasons:

    - It is an uncommon occurrence, and the diagnosis can be missed. I identify one or two a year that has not been picked up by radiology. I do have the advantage of talking to the patient and knowing which nerve is in question by the location of the pain. The radiological findings can also be very subtle with the only indication being less fat around the nerve root.

- Many spine surgeons are not familiar with the technique of approaching this disc rupture from outside the spinal canal, which is the simplest procedure. If you should find yourself with this problem, try to find out if this is an option for your surgeon. Many will gravitate towards performing a fusion, which may not be necessary. The question to ask is, "Do you perform extraforaminal disc excisions?"

Difficult to See Extraforaminal Disc Rupture

I saw one patient who had severe pain down his right leg along the front of his thigh, which is a classic 4th lumbar nerve root pattern L4 pattern. He had seen several physicians, and no one could tell him why he was in so much pain, even though he had undergone an MRI. Injections, physical therapy, medications, and time had not helped. He was in severe pain for six weeks and no one had made a definitive diagnosis. He was not functioning well at work and was worried about losing his job.

After taking his history, I knew that it was the L4 nerve root by the location of the pain and that it was going to be a problem in the foramen (intraforaminal) or outside it (extraforaminal) since he had pain only when standing. Standing causes these areas to narrow and increase the pressure on the nerve. The only finding on the MRI was a slight decrease in the amount of fat surrounding the L4 nerve in the extraforaminal area between the 4th and 5th vertebra. After performing an extraforaminal disc excision at that specific spot, he was pain free within two weeks.

Knee or Spine Pain?

Pain solely in the kneecap is usually caused by softening cartilage in the patella (kneecap)—a common condition called chondromalacia patellae. However, pain in the kneecap can also be a sign of a rare situation where the 3rd lumbar nerve root is pinched. The path of this nerve is down the front of the thigh and stops at the knee. However, only the patellar area may hurt. Then, the knee may be treated without considering a spinal source of the pain.

I have evaluated several patients with this pattern of knee pain, who had first undergone arthroscopic knee surgery that (naturally) didn't work. The unsuccessful procedure didn't constitute a major disaster, but it was certainly a waste of money with some additional risk to the patient.

Why a Ruptured Disc is Usually Structural

Pain, weakness, numbness, tingling and burning are all symptoms consistent with a structural problem. A patient with a ruptured (herniated) disc and symptoms along the path of the affected nerve has a structural problem that is amenable to surgery. *Even so, it does not mean that surgery must be done.* It means only that surgery is an option if the pain is severe and/or prolonged enough to undergo the risks. Other factors, such as stress, sleep, physical conditioning, and medications also enter into the decision and are discussed chapter 5.

If the herniation weren't causing pressure on nerves or the spinal cord, it would not be considered structural, regardless of the pain or neurological patterns. Then it would be critical to look for other non-spine sources of the symptoms. Many times, I have seen unsuccessful spine surgery performed and a more serious diagnosis missed. Some of these included: bladder cancer in the pelvis, polymyalgia rheumatica, and ALS (Lou Gehrig's Disease).

Surgical Emergencies: Massive Disc Ruptures

There are a few emergent surgical scenarios that may occur as the result of large or massive disc ruptures. In the lower back, the most severe form this takes is called the *cauda equina syndrome,* which is described in Chapter 3. This is a true surgical emergency. Return of function is unpredictable but felt to be better with early surgery.

When a large central disc rupture occurs in the neck or thoracic spine the situation is even more emergent, because spinal cord tissue is less resilient. The constellation of symptoms is called *myelopathy,* also discussed in Chapter 3. If an acute disc rupture causes cord compression, it is an emergency, with even a less predictable return of function.

When is a Ruptured Disc Non-structural?

Frequently, a disc may be herniated in a spot that doesn't compress or irritate a nerve, or it is too small to cause a problem. Generally, there is no radicular pain, weakness or numbness because there is not much compression of the neurological structures.

There are several situations where a patient has degenerated discs with some leg or arm pain, but I am unable to make a straightforward diagnosis (Non-structural Type II). This is the case when radicular pain is vague and moves around. It's possible that the ambiguous pain is coming from the soft tissues around the hip, irritation of the band of tissue going down the side of the leg called the iliotibial band (IT band), the rotator cuff, tight trapezius muscle or any number of soft tissue imbalances in the upper or lower extremities. If there is minimal compression around the corresponding nerves to the painful area down the extremity, then surgery isn't an option. The difficulty arises when some significant, but not severe, compression might be causing the symptoms, and the decision to have surgery is not black-and-white.

It is fairly common to encounter a patient with a specific nerve that is painful but without an abnormality in the spine that explains the pain. In these situations, I would pursue extensive diagnostic testing. First, I would obtain a myelogram, followed by a CAT scan to avoid missing a problem in the spine. In a myelogram, an iodine dye is injected directly into the spinal canal, and the radiologist can observe the flow of the dye past the area in question. If the dye flows by freely, even if there is some constriction, surgery probably will not contribute to the solution.

Other possible sources should be considered, including shingles, tumors of the pelvis, sciatic nerve, or spinal cord; neurologic disorders such as ALS (Lou Gehrig's disease) and others presented in Chapter 3. You may not uncover the explanation for the pain, but you will have ruled out serious problems. If the workup is negative, I call the condition primary lumbar radiculitis, which means that the nerve is irritated without a known cause. There are drugs to treat the symptoms, and after a period of time the pain usually goes away. This is another example where surgery is not a solution if there is no identifiable lesion.

Patients with severe neck or low back pain can have pain that is *referred* to the legs. In other words, they are experiencing leg pain but there is no evidence of a specific nerve pattern of pain that I would call radicular. This pain starts in the small nerve fibers arranged in a web-like configuration in the muscles around the spine that exist in the envelope of tissue called the fascia. Just like the ripples from a rock dropped in a pond, the pain impulses can travel into the fascial tissues in the upper leg. In these cases, I would *never* consider surgery; instead it's best to pursue rehab of the soft tissues.

3. Spinal Stenosis

Spinal stenosis is narrowing of the spinal canal from any cause, including tumor, fracture, infection, congenital defects, disc ruptures, or degeneration. This section will refer only to degenerative spinal stenosis, which is by far the most common type.

Spinal stenosis due to degeneration develops gradually over years. Firm, hard tissues such as bone spurs, enlarged facet joints, buckled discs, or the *ligamentum flavum* (between the lamina at the back of the spine) circumferentially narrow the central canal and compress neurological tissues. Although symptoms may come and go, the constriction will never improve, resulting in strictures that resemble the narrow part of an hourglass.

Narrowing from progressive degeneration can occur in three other areas:

1.   Where the nerve leaves the spinal canal (*recess stenosis*)

2.   In the foramen (bony canal on the side of the spine surrounding the exiting nerve

3.   Outside the foramen

Constrictions in these three areas cause only radicular symptoms, never myelopathy, because only peripheral nerves are located here.

The cause of degenerative stenosis isn't known. While all people have some degeneration of their discs, most don't have stenosis.

But for those who do, between the enlarging facets, bulging discs, and thickening ligament, the spinal canal can become very tight.

Normally, the central lumbar spinal canal is about 15 mm in diameter (a little over half an inch) and the cervical canal is around 12 mm (a little under half an inch). Problems arise depending on the level of the spine where constriction occurs. In the neck, or cervical area, the spinal cord occupies most of the central canal, so symptoms occur when the diameter decreases to 8 or 9 mm. The lumbar spine has a good deal of cerebrospinal fluid (CSF) round the nerves, so the constriction can be as severe as 5—6 mm without symptoms. The same is true about the thoracic central canal: There is a lot more CSF around it than there is in the cervical spine. Therefore, degenerative thoracic myelopathy is uncommon compared to cervical myelopathy.

Structural Degenerative Spinal Stenosis

The problem is structural if the compression is severe enough to cause corresponding radicular or mylopathic symptoms.

Cervical and Thoracic Stenosis

In the central cervical and thoracic spinal canal, the narrowing must be severe enough that the bony and ligamentous tissues must make direct contact with the spinal cord in order to be considered the cause of symptoms. If there is still cerebrospinal fluid around the spinal cord, there is not direct pressure on the neurological tissues. Often the cord will be deformed by the severity of the compression. The symptoms will be some combination of the myelopathic symptoms mentioned in Chapter 3. Myelopathy can be caused by other abnormalities besides tissue compression, so if there are any questions about the source of symptoms, a more complete neurological workup is mandatory.

In the cervical spine, foraminal stenosis will create radicular symptoms such as pain and weakness of a muscle, and occasionally a combination of symptoms. Thoracic radiculopathy is rare; but when it occurs, it presents a burning pain that surrounds the rib cage. Of course, the pain pattern must match the abnormal anatomy if it is to be amenable to surgery.

Another example of a non-spine cause of upper extremity symptoms is carpal tunnel syndrome (CTS), which is often confused with a 6th cervical foraminal compression, since they both travel down the thumb side of the hand. It's possible for a patient to have both.

Lumbar Stenosis

The lumbar spine is the most common location for degenerative stenosis. It occurs more in females; and L3-4 and L4-5 levels are most commonly affected. The lowest level, L5-S1 is rarely involved. Why lumbar stenosis occurs is unknown. Some people are born with huge spinal canals and it is almost impossible to develop enough constriction to compress the nerves. Others are born with small canals, a condition called *congenital spinal stenosis*; and nerve compression can occur even with relatively mild anatomical abnormalities.

In order for lumbar stenosis to be considered a structural problem, the constriction must be tight enough that there is no fluid around the nerves. Otherwise, the nerves are not being pinched; there is just less fluid. This may sound obvious to you, but a lot of surgery is performed to relieve pressure that doesn't exist.

The overall success rate for relieving pain and improving function is only about 65% (Herno). It would seem that if compression were the problem, then surgery to relieve it should have a higher success rate. Reasons for failure include performing an inadequate decompression, failing to address the constriction in the foramen or outside it, and destabilizing the spine.

The second requirement to consider lumbar stenosis a structural problem is that the pattern of symptoms must match the level where the constriction is taking place. We have already seen that nerve compression is not a cause of axial pain. But the symptoms created by lumbar stenosis down the leg(s) are usually quite vague and widespread. This is one scenario that is an exception: The symptoms do not need to perfectly match the structural abnormality. Here is a list of the range of symptoms.

- Diffuse aching or burning—may travel around

- Legs feeling "rubbery" or slightly numb

- Legs fatiguing when walking—the tighter the stenosis, the shorter the walking distance before having symptoms.

- Symptoms worse when standing and walking, promptly relieved by sitting or bending forward. Many people lean on shopping carts while at a store, giving rise to the term, "the shopping cart sign."

- Severe muscle weakness or bowel and bladder dysfunction are late symptoms and the compression must be severe to be considered the source.

The cardinal pattern of symptoms is that they are worse when standing or walking and better or absent when sitting. It is postulated that the ligaments at the back of the lamina (ligamentum flavum) thicken when upright and narrow when stretched in the sitting position.

Similar symptoms can result from vascular insufficiency, from poor blood supply to the legs. In that case, however, the symptoms worsen with walking and lessen with standing still. With lumbar stenosis, symptoms are worse than sitting both while standing or walking. If the pain were worse with sitting, I'd look for another cause. If the diffuse leg symptoms are constant regardless of position, it usually means the constriction is extreme or there is another problem that is being missed.

Non-structural Degenerative Spinal Stenosis

In order for spinal stenosis to be considered a structural problem, the constriction must be severe enough to cause compression on the spinal cord (myelopathy) or peripheral nerves (radiculopathy).

Pinched nerves do not cause axial pain; therefore, axial pain is not relieved by surgery intended to decompress nerves. Patients often cancel surgery once they understand the goal is only to relieve distal radicular symptoms, and not their axial pain. If the radiculopathy or myelopathy requires surgery, the axial pain will not disappear—in fact, it can be made worse.

Ongoing neck or back pain after spine surgery is possibly the most common complaint I have encountered over my career. If you go through the ordeal of spine surgery expecting it to relieve your neck, thoracic, or low back pain, only to discover that it didn't, your emotional reaction is likely to aggravate your pain.

Unhappy Surgical Outcome Because of Ongoing Back Pain

A turning point in my surgical decision-making occurred many years ago with a patient in her mid-forties who had a central spinal stenosis causing bilateral pain down the front sides of both of her legs. The pain was worse with standing and walking and relieved by sitting. It was a classic structural problem. She was also experiencing axial low back pain worse than the radicular pain. She adamantly refused to engage in any part of the rehab program, and at that time I didn't insist on it. I saw her every two to three weeks over a six-month period, without significant improvement in either her back or leg pain. I clearly told her that surgery would not relieve her back pain but usually improves leg symptoms. After many conversations, she convinced me that, if surgery improved her leg pain, she would participate in the rehab. I performed a simple decompression at one level of her lumbar spine, which completely resolved her leg pain. However, her back pain worsened (often the case without rehab), and she was furious. Reminding her of our pre-operative conversations only escalated her anger, and she once again refused to participate in rehab or any non-operative care. After another six months of working to convince her to try almost anything, she quit coming to see me. My whole team subsequently pointed out that patients who actively engaged in some form of a structured care program consistently did better; and they asked me to stop performing elective surgery if a patient didn't want to assume responsibility for that portion of his or her own care. I did, and that simple decision transformed my practice. Our surgical outcomes became much more consistent, and many patients cancelled surgery because their both their back and leg pain resolved from their participation in the structured care program.

4. Spondylolisthesis

"Spondylo-" means vertebra and "listhesis" is a medical term for "slip," so spondylolisthesis means slippage of the vertebra. Specifically, it is slippage of one vertebra onto the vertebra below it. There are five types of slippage:

- Degenerative—caused by the degeneration eroding the facets and allowing the slippage

- Isthmic—About 5% of the adult population has a boney defect in a lamina so that the back of vertebra is not attached to the front.

- Congenital –Born with abnormalities of the lamina, pedicles, or vertebral bodies that cause the respective level to be weaker.

- Traumatic—A high-energy trauma can separate the front from the back of the spine and create a severe instability.

- Pathological—Tumors can destroy and destabilize the spinal column.

Only the first two will be discussed, as the last three are rare. Spondylolisthesis is often cited as a reason for performing surgery; but I contend that in many cases the surgery is unnecessary if the spine is stable.

Degenerative Spondylolisthesis

Of the different causes of slippage, degeneration of the vertebral segment (defined as vertebrae-disc-vertebrae) is the most common. The process includes the whole cross-section of a given level, including the discs, vertebral bodies, ligaments and the joints in the back of the spine, called *facets*. All the relationships change between the vertebrae. Usually the vertebra settle down on each other and remain aligned. However, the abnormal anatomy can cause the upper vertebrae to slide forward, and this is what is called degenerative spondylolisthesis. Less often, the upper vertebra slides backwards, but still is called a degenerative spondylolisthesis. The direction it slides is not a factor in surgical decision-making.

The majority of degenerative slips occur in the lumbar spine (lower back), but the problem can also occur in the cervical region. With the rib cage stabilizing most of the thoracic spine, spondylolisthesis there is rare. The decision whether to repair the slippage surgically is based on two considerations:

1. Is the area of the slippage stable or unstable?

2. Is there an associated stenosis (narrowing) of the central canal or foraminal area severe enough to trap nerves or the spinal cord?

Stable vs. unstable

- Stable: Our bodies respond to wear and tear as well as inflammation by forming bone spurs. The exact reason is unclear, but it is consistent. Most of these are harmless and add stability to a given joint by a buttress effect. Bone spurs become problematic when they encroach on vital structures. For example, massive bone spurs originating from the front of the spine rarely cause symptoms because there is so much space in the abdomen. The spine also becomes more stable regardless of alignment because of the larger surface area. When the facet joints at the back of the spine enlarge, there is a higher chance that they will encroach on neurological structures, since they are in closer proximity to them. Often there is enough compression that nerve or spinal cord symptoms result, but this also adds stability to the segment. A stable spine, regardless of the alignment, is not a cause of axial pain.

- Unstable: A less common scenario is that the wear and tear erodes and destroys the facet joints, causing spurs to form and make the spine less stable. The extra motion causes more erosion and more instability. There is excessive motion between the vertebrae between bending forward and backwards as measured on an x-ray. Most surgeons consider motion of four or more millimeters to be a structural problem and a possible source of pain.

Associated stenosis

Degenerative spondylolisthesis can occur without any narrowing of the spinal canal, or it can create constriction of the neurological structure in the middle of the canal as they exit the side of the spine. Central canal constriction in the neck and thoracic spine compresses the spinal cord and can cause neurological symptoms called *myelopathy*; now, pain is less of an issue. Since the spinal cord ends at the level of the first lumbar vertebrae, at the top of the lower back, central stenosis of the lumbar spine will cause only radicular symptoms of one or several nerve roots. Here, pain is more of an issue in the surgical decision-making.

Nerves compressed after they leave the spinal cord create only radicular symptoms, with pain being a more common decision point than neurological compromise. Nerves can be impinged just before they exit the canal (recess stenosis), in the openings on the side of the spine (foraminal stenosis), or after they leave the foramen (extraforaminal stenosis).

Narrowing or stenosis can occur in the presence of a stable *or* unstable spondylolisthesis, but there is additional trauma to the nerves and/or cord with the extra motion. In other words, neurological symptoms can occur with less constriction. Furthermore, the irritation from the motion often seems to be associated with a layer of inflammatory tissue directly adherent to the nerves. Surgery is more challenging in that it is difficult to peel this tissue off to relieve the pressure. There is a greater risk of inadvertently entering the dural sac (the sac of fluid protecting the nerves) with a resultant leakage of cerebrospinal fluid.

Degenerative Spondylolisthesis as a Structural Issue (Type I)

Spondylolisthesis is a structural problem when the following conditions are present:

- Enlarged tissues (bones, ligaments, discs) are narrowing the spinal canal to the extent that no CSF is protecting the nerves or spinal cord and there are corresponding neurological findings and/or matching pain patterns in the arms or legs.

- If there are radicular or myelopathic symptoms, the level can be stable or unstable.

- Matching the leg or arm symptoms with the level of compression is usually a straightforward process; often, there's just one level of slippage and the rest of the spine is normal.

- When there is *only* axial pain, diagnosing degenerative spondylolisthesis as the pain source is not as clear; but evidence includes:

  - A large gap in the facet joints

  - A buildup of fluid in the facet joints

  - Excessive motion of more than 4 mm forward and backward in the low back and 2—3 mm in the neck

It is difficult to "match" the lesion with axial symptoms even with extra motion. It's helpful if only one level is unstable.

Unstable Spine and Avoided Surgery

Years ago I encountered a woman in her fifties whose case really drove this point home. An avid runner, she had been experiencing LBP for over a year, without a clear-cut cause. Her x-rays showed a degenerative spondylolisthesis that moved 1 cm with flexion and extension of her spine. This was the most unstable degenerative spondylolisthesis I had ever seen. I assumed that I would be performing a one-level fusion. But her MRI scan did not reveal any nerve compression and she had no leg pain. When I explained the surgical procedure to her, she simply didn't want to do it. After about six months of physical therapy and working out at the gym, her back pain disappeared.

Degenerative Spondylolisthesis as a Non-structural Issue (Type II)

When the spondylolisthesis consists of a simple mal-alignment without excessive motion, it's not a cause of axial pain. On the surface, this seems obvious since hardly anyone's spine is perfectly aligned. However, I have evaluated an endless number of patients who have had their stable, "mal-aligned" spines fused for back pain, without relief. A fusion is intended to stabilize an unstable spine.

Facets often enlarge to the point where they practically fuse the segment spontaneously. It is described as an "auto-fusion." Enlarged facets may pinch nerves and cause leg or arm pain; but, as there is little motion, the vertebral segment would not be considered a source of *axial* pain.

In another instance, as the vertebrae slip, the disc can completely disappear, and a bony bridge can form across the disc space. This "auto-fusion" creates a *more* stable segment. Thus, it would never be considered the cause of axial pain. Nonetheless, such a "collapsed disc" is frequently cited as a reason to perform a spine fusion—especially if it is misaligned.

Isthmic Spondylolisthesis

The *laminae* are flat bony structures that protect the back of the spinal canal and are located between the facet joints. Similar to shingles on a roof, one appears on each level of the spine. The *pars* is the area on the sides of each lamina that spans the space between the facet joints and supports the back of the spine. The bone is noticeably thicker and stronger. The nerves pass immediately under the pars, so it is an important landmark in surgery. About 5% of the adult population has a bony defect in this are called a *pars defect.* There is less bony support and the front and back of the spine are not connected at that level. At surgery, we see that the lamina is loose and "floating," It sounds dangerous, but the main role of the facets and lamina is not support but rather to keep the spine aligned. Over 80% of the strength is from the front of the spine. The most common affected level is L5-S1, followed by L4-5. This condition is called an isthmic spondylolisthesis.

These defects allow the affected vertebra to slide forward while the back part doesn't move and lamina is left behind. So, the vertebrae can slip all of the way off of the lower vertebra without damaging any nerves. This is possible because the central canal opens up and enlarges. With the pars defect, the lamina never causes constriction in the central canal. The severity of the slip is graded in the following manner whether or not the level is stable.

- Spondylolysis—Only a bony defect at the pars without any slippage
- Grade 1—Upper vertebra slipped up to 25% of the width of the lower vertebra.
- Grade 2—up to 50% slip
- Grade 3—up to 75%
- Grade 4—up to 100%
- Grade 5—the upper vertebra has slipped and fallen off the lower vertebra. Believe it or not, this often happens without any nerves being pinched enough to cause pain or neurological deficits. Another term for this condition is *spondyloptosis*.

Isthmic Spondylolisthesis as a Structural Issue

Similar to degenerative spondylolisthesis, when a slipped vertebra compresses a nerve, causing leg pain in the pattern of that nerve, it's a structural problem. The narrowing around the nerves occurs only in the foramen as the nerves are exiting the spinal canal. Since this condition often appears in younger patients who have spines that are otherwise normal, there is little guesswork in determining which level is the culprit.

In these cases, the pain is commonly in one or both legs when the patient is standing or walking. The foramen opens while sitting. In a normal spine there is enough space to accommodate the narrowing that occurs with standing or walking, but with isthmic spondylolisthesis the narrowing is severe enough that the symptoms occur almost instantly. The affected levels and their corresponding nerves and pain patterns are:

- L5-S1: L5 nerve root down the side of the leg; occasionally down the back of the leg
- L4-5: L4 nerve root down the front of the leg; occasionally down the side of the leg
- L3-4: L3 nerve root in the groin and to the knee; occasionally down the front of the leg

With only axial pain (in the absence of radicular pain), it's more difficult to place isthmic spondylolisthesis into a structural category. If the patient's LBP is consistently worse with standing and better with sitting, the pars defect may be the source of the pain. While injections are sometimes used to pinpoint an area as the pain generator, there is little evidence to support that test as a valid diagnostic tool, being that it is highly subjective.

I would consider an isthmic spondylolisthesis a possible structural low back pain generator where there is excessive motion between the vertebrae. Generally, it would be more than 3 mm of motion between the vertebrae while flexing and extending the spine, under x-ray observation. The movement can be dramatic. My impression is that this amount of motion *does* contribute to LBP.

Isthmic Spondylolisthesis as a Non-Structural Issue

Without leg pain or excessive motion, isthmic spondylolisthesis is a non-structural diagnosis. Even in a more severe slip, when the disc is completely collapsed and immobile, it would not be considered a source of pain, since it is stable. Should a patient have a pars defect but no vertebral slippage, it is called *spondylolysis*, a bony defect of the lamina on the back of the spine. It's common for the disc at this level to be completely normal or just slightly degenerated; in other words, probably not a pain generator.

Some patients with isthmic spondylolisthesis have leg pain, suggesting that the slippage might be the source; but if an MRI reveals abundant fat around the nerve roots, there is no nerve compression, and therefore it is not the problem. Other causes of leg pain should be considered.

I have observed many fusions performed on stable pars defects for low back pain, although that procedure has little chance of working. The patients are often under 30 years old, which means they have a lifetime of adjacent-level breakdowns to look forward to, in addition to a continuation of the original pain.

In my experience, patients do poorly having ongoing back pain after undergoing a fusion for a stable spondylolisthesis. I have long somewhat lightly said that the biggest risk of having an isthmic spondylolysis or spondylolisthesis is having a surgeon discover it and perform a fusion. Bur this is no joke. I saw this occur multiple times throughout my career. *If you do not have gross instability associated with the pars defect, do not consider a fusion for back pain.*

The Disc, Not the Spondylolysis, was the Pain Generator

During my first year in practice, when I was liberally performing fusions for discogenic low back pain and spondylolysis, I treated Pat, a twenty-five-year-old with persistent low back pain. Tests revealed disc degeneration at L4-5 and L5-S1 and also a pars defect at L5-S1, but without slippage or instability. I had him do rehab in the form of physical therapy and back education with consistent attention to good posture and body mechanics for six months; but the back pain persisted, so I decided to perform a fusion at L5-S1, which was significantly degenerated in addition to the pars defect. I felt the combination of the degeneration and the pars defect at this lowest level was enough reason to proceed.

About two weeks before the scheduled fusion, he ruptured his disc between the fourth and fifth vertebrae (L4-5). In the pre-rupture phase of a disc herniation, there is usually a lot of pain and spasm from the ring around the irritated disc. When the ring breaks, and the pressure is relieved, the back pain resolves. His back pain disappeared, but he developed pain in a classic L5 pattern down the side of his left leg. The fifth nerve root was pinched and irritated by the L4-5 disc herniation.

I now faced a difficult decision. I was routinely performing fusions for back pain at the time, so I strongly considered a two-level fusion; but I decided on a simple disc excision at L4-5. Pat had a smooth recovery and no residual back or leg pain. Twenty-seven years later, his back problem never returned.

In retrospect, I can now see that the L5-S1 level was not the cause of his pain; rather, it was a result of the L4-5 disc in a pre-rupture state. So, not only would the fusion have been ineffective; it would have placed even more stress on L4-5. Furthermore, if I'd performed the originally planned one-level L5-S1 fusion, Pat would have quickly needed a second operation to fuse L4-5, as it was a compromised disc. One simple discectomy versus two lumbar fusions: Pat's case was my first hint that fusions for back pain might not be the best choice.

A Damaging Fusion for a Lumbar Strain

George, a middle-aged gentleman, was applying for work with a government agency that required some physical tests as part of the application process. During one such test he fell and severely twisted his back. Given his history and immediate onset of lower back pain, George's diagnosis was a lumbar strain.

His x-rays revealed normal discs at every level and a stable spondylolysis at L5-S1 (the lowest level of the spine). Six weeks after the injury, a surgeon at a major center recommended that he undergo an L5-S1 fusion for ongoing LBP.

This surgeon inserted the L5 screw on the right too far towards the canal and pierced the 5th lumbar nerve root. He woke with extreme leg pain, and the screw was removed the next day after a CAT scan revealed the misplaced screw.

When he saw me six months later, his leg pain was still extreme and the fusion had not healed, although it was stable. I did not recommend further surgery, as there was no ongoing pressure on the nerve; surgery would neither affect the leg pain nor help the back pain. The nerve damage was permanent. He was understandably angry and did not want to hear about any of the other options available to decrease his pain without surgery. He found another surgeon to re-do the fusion—with no relief of his pain.

Improper placement of a screw is an ongoing unfortunate complication. With modern nerve monitoring and x-rays, it occurs less frequently; but the incidence is still 5 - 10% (Goz, Fritzell). While complications are universally accepted risks of any surgery, in George's case it could have been completely avoided, because his surgery was unnecessary. His muscular strain would have completely resolved over three to six months with an organized rehab program. The spondylolysis, an incidental discovery, was stable. There were no indications for surgery at all.

In terms of the Treatment Grid, George entered the medical system as a IIB patient: No identifiable source of pain, and angry at the agency, whom he felt caused his injury. After surgery, he moved to the IB category, even more upset, now that he was worse off, with a surgically weakened spine and a permanently damaged nerve.

This is just one of many cases where a patient had an operation that was not indicated, for a stable spondylolysis. Prior to surgery George had been an active and productive person. This is one of the reasons he was so enraged and desperate. Before the surgery he had absolutely no limitations on his full life. But he suffered a major, permanent complication that will affect the rest of his life, undergoing a procedure with an unacceptable benefit-to-risk ratio. The other obvious issue is that he had been in pain for only six weeks; surgery should have never part of the discussion.

5. Spinal Deformity

The word "deformity" has an ominous sound that implies a serious problem. However, while deformities can cause problems, they are usually inconsequential. No spine is perfectly straight—most are slightly misaligned or curved. Only when the magnitude of a curve is greater than ten degrees as measured from the top and bottom of the curve does a patient even receive a deformity diagnosis.

The curve is measured by computing the largest angle from the top of its upper vertebra to the bottom of its lowest vertebra, with a seven-degree margin of error. For example, if an x-ray revealed an angle measuring 38 degrees, and four months later it was re-measured on a new x-ray as 43 degrees (5 degrees difference), we would conclude that the curve had not progressed. If you are contemplating surgery based on whether your curve is progressing, make sure the same levels are measured each time and the same surgeon does the measuring throughout the progression study. As each physician has his or her own way of drawing the lines and measuring them, a great source of inaccuracy is having different doctors marking the studies.

Most of the time, the spine compensates for abnormal curvatures with changes in other parts of the spine, the pelvic angle, or in the hips. The goals of all the normal curves of the spine is to keep your head centered directly over the center of your pelvis with minimal muscle tension required to maintain it. The deformity is considered *compensated* if your head is within five centimeters of the center in any direction. If the head is greater than five centimeters away from pelvic center, it is considered an unbalanced or *decompensated* deformity.

Evaluating whether a deformity is balanced or decompensated is measured on full-length standing x-rays with the knees locked straight. Normally, the base of your neck is centered directly over the back your sacrum; a plumb line drawn from the seventh cervical vertebra will intersect the sacrum. In a decompensated scoliosis (sideways curvature) that line will be off to the side, and in kyphosis (bent forward), the line will be in front of the sacrum.

Young patients can more easily compensate problem areas in their spines than can older patients because they are much more flexible. For example, if a seventeen-year-old patient has a compression deformity from a fracture, we can expect his spine to adjust its overall alignment in order to re-center his or her head over the pelvis. But a stiffer, 70-year-old spine loses much of this ability to compensate.

General Deformity Principles

The key issue in adult deformity is whether or not your head is centered over your pelvis. In my practice, the one symptom that drove patients to consider major deformity surgery was if they were tilted forward, unable to stand up straight without bending their knees. It is difficult to fully engage in activities of everyday life while you are tolerating a pitched-forward posture.

Patients with scoliosis should be aware that a curve in their spine, regardless of its size, isn't necessarily a source of back pain (Nachemson). A curve can increase while the head remains balanced over the pelvis: It progresses directly downward, or *telescopes*. The indications for performing a fusion based on the size of the curve have not been defined in the literature. There is high major complication rate and the benefits do not outweigh the risks. What's more, the research hasn't documented the effectiveness of surgery compared to a well-orchestrated rehab program.

There is usually a lot of bone spurring with adult spinal deformities. These arthritic segments hardly move. The body creates them in order to stabilize the spine and stop the curve from progressing. It is also logical to conclude that less motion leads to less pain. We use the term "arthritis" to describe these spurs, but they are much different than the arthritis of a constantly moving joint, such as your knee or hip.

If your curved spine contains severely narrowed discs, some surgeons consider them a source of pain. Since the data reveals little if any correlation between degenerated discs and low back pain (Jarvik, Boden), it isn't logical to believe a greater number of them would be a source of pain.

Types of Deformity

The two most common types of spinal deformity are *scoliosis*, a sideways curve in the shape of an S or a C; and *kyphosis*, a forward curve of the spine. When both deformities are present in the same person, the condition is called *kyphoscoliosis*.

Scoliosis

Scoliosis usually occurs from 1) rotation of the spinal column or 2) sideways collapse of the spine, 3) both rotation and collapse.

Rotation of the Spinal Column

Infantile, congenital, juvenile, and adolescent scoliosis are some of the deformities that occur in young patients before their growth plates have closed, when their skeletons are considered skeletally immature. After skeletal maturity, scoliosis is considered an adult deformity, because there is less of a chance of the curve becoming worse after growth has stopped. Pre-adult deformities are permanent and can progress. The presence of these pre-existing curves makes the decision-making difficult later in life.

One factor of interest to surgeons is that some of these deformities are caused by rotation of the spinal column. As the column twists, it moves sideways, creating a curve—possibly two or three. Whether these curves are addressed surgically in childhood or adulthood, the rotational component makes the surgery technically challenging because the anatomy is especially distorted. Straightening and stabilizing the curve requires placing screws down the pedicles that connect the back and front of the spine. Normally, the anatomical landmarks are clear, and the screws are placed in a fairly consistent manner directly into the spine. But if the curve is rotated, the angle of approach is different at every level and requires more time and x-rays for accurate placement. Vital vascular and neurological structures are at risk when the screws are placed outside the pedicles.

The most common curve prior to adulthood is called *idiopathic* scoliosis, meaning "unknown." They usually become apparent around ages eight to ten and progress during the child's growth years. The progression usually stops after the child stops growing— in girls about 18 months after the onset of their menses; in boys, potentially into their late teens. For reasons that are unclear, clinically significant progression is more common in girls, meaning that more interventions are needed to prevent future problems. For example, bracing to halt progression is recommended when the scoliosis is greater than 25 degrees; and surgery to fuse the curve is considered after it reaches 45 to 50 degrees. In adulthood, these numbers become less important because the chances of the curve becoming worse are much lower.

The goal of treatment, whether it is bracing, exercises or surgery, is a curve less than 45 degrees by the time the child stops growing. Living with a curve of this magnitude presents no physical limitations or medical consequences in adulthood. In younger patients, curves rarely decompensate because there is so much flexibility that allows the head to remain balanced over the pelvis.

Since it has been documented that adolescent idiopathic curves of more than 30 degrees may progress in adulthood, most surgeons will recommend follow up x-rays to monitor any significant progression.

Sideways Collapse

When the spinal column collapses sideways, there is usually some rotation as well; but rotation is not the driving force behind this form of scoliosis. Rather, the origins for sideways-collapsing scoliosis include congenital (birth defect), neuromuscular (disease such as polio or cerebral palsy), post-traumatic condition after a serious fracture, and progressive degeneration of the spine.

Degeneration occurs in the discs and the facet joints, and if it happens on one side more than the other, a sideways collapse results. If it occurs on one or two levels, it called *segmental collapse*, and the deformity is minimal. Symptoms occur if the collapse traps an exiting nerve, causing a radiculopathy. Should degeneration occur over multiple levels, there might be a scoliosis that is still balanced. There is a trend in spine surgery to consider the combination of deformity and degeneration as a source of axial pain; but there is no data to support that notion.

Degeneration is usually eventually present in other forms of scoliosis that cause larger deformities. But the origin and size of the curve is not as much of an issue as whether the deformity is a balanced or has decompensated.

Kyphosis

Kyphosis describes an abnormal forward curvature of the spine—"abnormal" defined by an angle greater than generally accepted norms. This varies with the location on the spinal column.

The curve in the spine that normally faces backward in the cervical and lumbar spine is called *lordosis*. The thoracic spine has a normal kyphosis between 40—50 degrees and is considered abnormal if it exceeds 55 degrees. There are a couple transition areas that are normally straight, between the cervical and thoracic spine and at the junction of the thorasic and lumbar spine. So, any changes in the spine that cause the straight sections to be bent forward, the kyphosis to exceed the norm, or less lordosis can be considered a relative kyphosis. For example, loss of lumbar lordosis is common as the discs degenerate and narrow in the front of the lumbar spine. At some point, this settling may cause your body to lean forwards. The term for this lumbar kyphosis (loss of lordosis) is *flatback syndrome.*

The net result of these curvatures is that the head is directly centered over the pelvis. When you are young, the spine is usually flexible enough to compensate for an abnormal area, to keep you balanced. Your spine continues to adapt as you age; but at some tipping point, if the deformity is too large, or the rest of the spine has become too stiff to compensate, your body will lean forward. Decompensated kyphosis is especially distressing due to the constant feeling of falling forward and the ongoing stress on lower back muscles trying to regain a balanced posture. These muscles were not intended to maintain that type of ongoing stress and will fatigue within minutes.

Kyphosis has many causes. Any process or injury that decreases the height of the vertebral bodies and/or discs in the *front* of the spine can create an abnormal kyphosis. The *back* of the spine remains unchanged, so there is an asymmetric shortening of the front of the spinal column.

One such condition that adversely affects any spinal deformity, in addition to causing one of its own, is osteoporosis. One of the tragedies of the 21st century is outliving your skeleton. The average life span in 1950 was only 47 years, while today in the US it is 78. This is largely a result of antibiotics, which are considered to have added twenty years to average life spans, and cardiovascular advances, which have added another ten. The upshot of this, though, is that after around age 45, calcium loss becomes an issue, especially in women. There is an increasingly higher incidence of osteoporosis (soft bones) in the aging population. Patients with osteoporosis can experience multiple compression fractures and develop significant deformities. If a deformity is already present, osteoporosis can make it worse. It can happen quickly, and the deformity is often severe in potentially any direction. *Take your calcium daily!*

You have probably seen the classic "hunchback" kyphosis when the curve is in the upper thoracic spine; in the lower spine the whole upper body pitches forward. As uncomfortable as the hunchback posture looks, it usually causes little pain. The muscular stress in the lower back caused by kyphosis, however, is usually uncomfortable because so much sustained muscle force is required to stand upright. A term used to describe this unfortunate condition is *flatback syndrome.*

Another frequent cause of kyphosis in adults is progressive disc degeneration. In a normal spine, the discs play an important role in creating the curve in the lower back. As discs degenerate and collapse with age, they are unable to maintain this curve. The stiffer adult spine doesn't allow other parts of the spine to adjust and maintain overall balance. As you are pitched forwards, your soft tissues in the front of the hips shorten and limit your capacity to stand up even more. Since it takes more effort to stand up and walk, patients tend to sit more, again causing these tissues around the hips to contract even more. Stretching out the hip capsules and hip flexors can help somewhat but it takes an ongoing routine to maintain it. These tissues do become quite tight and are difficult to stretch. At some point, the patient pitches forward.

Back surgery can unwittingly cause kyphosis. Even a simple one-level fusion in a normal, straight spine has the potential to cause major problems over time. The stiff segment causes more forces to be concentrated above and below it, and over time can speed up degeneration and collapse of the adjacent discs. Longer fusions cause greater forces to be concentrated at the ends, increasing the chances of breakdown. The term for this problem is *junctional kyphosis,* and it occurs in about one in three patients with long fusions (Kim). The consequences of repeat surgeries, pain, and occasional neurological compromise are devastating.

Breakdown Around a Prior Fusion

Tom, a middle-aged patient in his fifties, was bent forward about 30 degrees and tilted to the right about 20 degrees when standing. He had lived that way for six years when he initially saw me. In the mid-1990s he had undergone a simple L4-5 laminectomy; and because of ongoing low back pain, he subsequently underwent a one-level L4-5 fusion. Within three years, his spine had collapsed both above and below the fusion, leaving him with a kyphosis of his lower back (flatback).

I performed a four-level fusion from L2 to the sacrum, using screws and rods to stabilize his spine. The operation corrected 80% of his deformity and markedly decreased his back pain; but he still required low dose narcotics and was moderately limited by the stiffness of his spine.

What if, instead of rushing into back surgery the first time around, Tom had first tried out an aggressive rehab program? Not only did he have an excellent chance of decreasing his pain to an acceptable level; learning stress management skills may have improved his overall quality of life as well. He certainly *never* would have developed his deformity. His is a classic story in that he had a structural problem (Type I) that was solved by a simple decompression. The ongoing back pain and disc degeneration is a non-structural (Type II) problem, and with ongoing pain (and frustration) he was probably a Type B. Operating on a Type IIB patient not only isn't effective, but patients are often made much worse. Tom developed a severe deformity and now was in the IB quadrant. He did respond to more surgery, but even with the extra rehab that we routinely do in a Type B patient, he wasn't able to regain the same function he would have if he had never undergone a fusion. This is one of the reasons I wrote Chapter 8 on how to avoid becoming a IB patient. If you start there, then it is just the way it is. However, there is no reason to end up there because of medical interventions.

It May Not Be the Spine

In the case of kyphosis, it is important to understand the origin of the imbalance. It may not be the spine. I have seen patients with severe hip arthritis who cannot stand up. This is because osteoarthritis creates bone spurs that limit hip motion, especially standing up. Then the soft tissues in the front of the hip shorten. The result of being tipped forward can be dramatic. The hip should always be addressed first with physical therapy, exercise, medications, and possibly surgery. A hip replacement is less risky than major adult deformity surgery.

The hips also may be a problem without arthritis. For example, prolonged sitting, such as being wheelchair-bound for years, creates severe contractures of the soft tissues in front of the hips, preventing the patient from being able to stand up straight. The treatment is aggressive rehab to stretch out the hip flexors; or, occasionally, surgery to release the contractures.

When patients with Parkinson's disease and other neuro-muscular diagnoses tend to tilt forward, aggressive rehab consisting of stretching and strengthening is always the first choice of treatment. First of all, the spinal deformity is often a lesser factor than the weakness and contractures. Secondly, if a major deformity surgery were to be performed, patients will usually tip back forward, negating the benefit from the surgery.

Spinal Deformity as a Structural Problem (Type I)

Several variables affect whether a spinal deformity can be considered a significant clinical problem. They are:

- A trunk imbalance severe enough that the patient feels like that they are always tipping forward or sideways.

- The magnitude of the curve is often cited as a reason for surgery. This is debatable.

- The presence of radicular symptoms, such as leg pain, numbness or weakness. While the pinched nerve would be structural, the deformity may not be the cause of axial pain. Axial pain and radicular symptoms have to be considered separately.

- Progression of the deformity over time

- Cardiopulmonary failure

- The curve or curves collapse when in the upright position compared to lying down.

Trunk Imbalance

Of all spinal deformities, the situation I most often addressed surgically was a trunk imbalance from kyphosis. In trying to compensate for being forced to look at the ground, patients usually had muscular neck pain as well as LBP. Besides, it is unpleasant to go through life in a bent-over position. Correcting such imbalances was one of the most challenging and rewarding experiences of my surgical practice.

In my pre-op conversations, I explained to my patients that I could generally obtain a good correction of their forward posture but was not sure about their axial pain. However, once the patient was upright, the muscles did not have to continually try to maintain balance. With full engagement of the DOC structured rehab concepts, including a full weight-training program, the back pain usually decreased dramatically. I felt it was not fusing the degenerated segments that resolved the pain; it was the combination of postural improvement and conditioning.

What was surprising to me was that I had several patients who had significant back pain from what I thought was decompensated deformities. To optimize the outcomes and minimize the complications, my protocol evolved to having all my deformity patients rehab for six more months before I considered surgery. Several patients actually stood up straight as their pain diminished and their strength improved. They cancelled their surgery. Many patients, once they had a significant decrease in pain and improvement in mood and function, decided that the deformity they had wasn't worth the risk of surgery to correct it; and they too cancelled surgery. During the last five years of my practice, I still saw many patients with significant deformities; but I operated on a much lower percentage of them.

Surgery to correct a trunk imbalance caused by scoliosis is a more difficult decision. Research has shown that this deformity, where the curve is sideways rather than forward, is better tolerated than a forward bend (Daubs). In my experience, the patients could not tell much difference in their posture after scoliosis surgery unless the correction of their decompensation had been dramatic. Neither is back pain as reliably relieved with surgery; since, unlike kyphosis and its forward tipping, scoliosis does not significantly stress the lower back muscles. If your main concern is tipping to one side, surgery might be a reasonable choice. But I would urge caution when considering it as a solution for LBP.

Magnitude of the Curve

With scoliosis, it's difficult to determine whether a balanced lumbar curve is the cause of low back pain, and the research is inconclusive. In the thoracic spine, it is less logical to consider scoliosis as a source of pain since it is so stable, being supported by the rib cage.

With kyphosis, there is a higher chance that a person can be pitched forwards to the point where it is unpleasant and painful. A normal spine is balanced with minimal muscular demands when standing upright, but your back muscles fatigue quickly when constantly working to straighten you up. So, the amount of decompensation is more of a factor in deciding on surgery than the magnitude of the kyphosis.

Severe kyphosis in the lower spine may compress the abdominal contents enough to create much discomfort, including the feeling of being "full" which becomes more important than the magnitude of the kyphosis. A large kyphosis creates more space for the heart and lungs, so cardiopulmonary issues are not a consideration when deciding about surgery. Many people with thoracic kyphosis are self-conscious about their "hunchback" appearance. It is a problem, but is it worth the risk of surgery? At least be clear in your own mind about why you are having the operation. Unfortunately, even with a dramatic correction, your body image may not change. Your opinion about your body is a memorized neurological circuit—just like phantom limb pain.

Severe Curve Without Limitations

A fifty-three-year-old woman came to see me to check on her scoliosis. She had worn a brace as a teenager for a 30-degree scoliosis in the middle part of her spine. She had not followed up on her spine for years and was curious as to how it looked. She jogged two to three miles at least three times a week and worked out regularly in the gym—and this was all to keep her tennis game competitive. She suffered neither back pain nor limitations from her scoliosis. We were both dismayed to discover that her lumbar curve had progressed to 84 degrees. What do you think I recommended? Nothing. How could I improve her life by subjecting her to ten hours of high-risk surgery, resulting in a stiff spine that would dramatically limit her lifestyle?

Deformity and Radicular Symptoms

Radicular pain in the presence of a spinal deformity can be an indicator of a structural (Type I) problem, but the deformity may or may not be the cause of the pain. Several conditions can cause the nerves to be compressed:

- One or two spinal segments can collapse on one side of the spine causing a small curvature that is technically a scoliosis. A better description would be "segmental collapse," since the rest of the spine usually compensates and remains balanced. It really isn't a true deformity.

- A prior, relatively large scoliosis (more than 30 degrees) may buckle at the apex of the curve. In this case, the scoliosis is part of the problem and considered structural if there is corresponding radicular pain or weakness.

- Spinal stenosis can develop at any point in a curve, but the deformity may or may not have caused it. If the constriction causes matching leg symptoms, it is a structural problem; the scoliosis should be considered separately.

- Kyphosis doesn't generally cause radicular symptoms because the foramen encasing the nerves opens as you lean forwards. However, when a kyphosis occurs in the thoracic or cervical spine from a fracture, tumor, or infection, the spinal cord may be compressed, causing neurologic deficits. That is definitely a structural issue that is often urgent or emergent.

The reason it is so critical to look at radicular pain and the deformity separately is that a much simpler surgery can often solve leg pain, with much less risk. The entire length of the curve(s) does not need to be fused.

Sciatica Selectively Solved in the Middle of a Scoliotic Curve

One of my patients, Don, was in his mid-fifties and an active mountain climber. Two years before I saw him, he had developed pain in the front of his left thigh that appeared while he was standing and walking. He had no back pain. Being determined, he continued to hike through the pain. It was a strain, however, and he'd begun to limit his walking.

His x-rays showed a significant scoliosis of around 55 degrees of his lumbar spine. The concave side of the curve had collapsed in the middle of his curve at L2-3 and L3-4 and was pushing on the L2 and L3 nerve roots. As these nerves travel to the front of the leg it was an exact match and clearly the source of his pain. When he stood up, the curve pushed even harder on the nerves. If I'd opted to correct the whole curve, it would have required that I fuse his spine from T10 (10th thoracic vertebra at the bottom of the rib cage) to the pelvis (eight levels). This is a high-risk procedure with significant blood loss and takes at least six hours. But it would relieve the compression on the nerves, because the foramina would have opened up as the spine straightened. After much discussion, we decided to just take the pressure off the nerves by performing a fusion at two levels, L2-3 and L3-4, without attempting to straighten the curve.

His leg pain was gone immediately after the operation and I was adamant that he remain inactive for four months so that the fusion could heal. At two-year follow-up he was back to full mountaineering activities with more awareness of body mechanics. He confessed to me on his last visit that he had been back in the mountains six weeks after the surgery.

Although x-rays showed that Don's fusion had healed nicely, his spine still looked "terrible." There was marked degeneration, bone spurs, and scoliosis above and below the fusion. But he had no low back pain. Although Don's scoliosis was factored into the surgical decision, it was a separate issue from the nerve compression. It was clear that a compressed nerve was the source of his pain; but his stable and balanced scoliosis did not need to be corrected. He may or not develop future problems with progressive scoliosis in the future, but it can be dealt with at that time.

Progression of Deformity Over Time

Spinal deformities have a much higher chance of increasing during a child's growth. At his time the tissues are more flexible and the curves create asymmetric pressure on the growth plates of the vertebrae. We have well-established guidelines that determine whether a deformity (scoliosis or kyphosis) should be simply observed, braced, or surgically stabilized. For example, in adolescent idiopathic scoliosis, the goal is to end up with a scoliosis of less than 50 degrees at skeletal maturity. The parameters for kyphosis are less well defined, and the cause of the deformity must be factored in. The goal for kyphosis treatment is to avoid a situation where the curve interferes with cardiopulmonary and musculoskeletal function and to prevent an unsightly deformity.

After the skeletal growth plates have closed, adults have a much lower chance of deformity progressing, but it still can. Factors that can contribute are: 1) The curve causing asymmetric forces that wear down the vertebrae and discs; 2) Osteoporosis that result in fractures and/or settling of the vertebral bodies; 3) Progressive neurological diseases resulting in increasing weakness and less trunk support; 4) Unknown reasons. However, progression of the curve in and of itself is not a reason to consider surgery, but it indicates that the deformity should be monitored with follow up x-rays. *The decisions around surgery should be made based only on the current problems created by it.* And remember, for a problem to be considered structural, it must cause corresponding symptoms.

It may seem like I am stating an obvious fact, but curve progression is often presented as a reason to perform surgery, even without any symptoms. For example, let's say you had a 35 degree scoliosis when you were twenty-five; and now, at age fifty, it is 55 degrees and balanced. You are having no pain or any physical limitations. How do we know that the progression didn't occur fifteen years ago and has been stable since? How do we know it is going to worsen? The only additional treatment that should be recommended is follow up x-rays according to your surgeon's judgment.

Cardiopulmonary Failure

Well-established data links the magnitude of a thoracic scoliotic curve with cardiopulmonary failure, caused by direct compression on the heart, large blood vessels, and lungs by the spine and rib cage. In these instances, the curve is usually over 80 degrees. Some deformities cause the thoracic spine to be bent backward, a condition we call *thoracic lordosis*. This bend causes a marked decrease in the distance between the sternum (breastbone) and the spine, reducing space for the blood vessels and heart. Lumbar curves, however, are not correlated with heart or lung failure.

The presence of any level of cardiopulmonary compromise with other causes being ruled out is a structural problem, even though the decision-making is not centered on pain or mobility. Unfortunately, these issues may be severe enough to preclude surgical intervention.

Increased kyphosis in the thoracic spine, while creating less room for the abdominal contents, opens up more space for the heart and lungs. So instead of affecting the heart and lungs, there may be a chronic feeling of being too full, and having a small appetite.

Collapsing Scoliosis

In collapsing scoliosis, multiple segments are unstable; and as we pointed out earlier in the chapter, excessive motion is generally considered a likely source of axial pain. In this uncommon scenario, the curve collapses and increases by more than 10 degrees by moving from a prone position to an upright one. Even though it may not result in a significant trunk imbalance, this degree of instability is a probable cause of pain.

Spinal Deformity as a Non-structural (Type II) Issue

A balanced deformity without instability, progression, or leg pain is *not* a problem warranting surgery. Spinal deformity should not be surgically treated if any of the following conditions are met:

- Balanced curves: Your head is centered over your pelvis.
- Stable curves: The deformity is stable as measured over time.
- Curve size alone

Balanced Curves

The human body has a remarkable ability to compensate for a deformity in one part of the spine by creating a "deformity" in another area of the spine. One common example is when excessive bending forward occurs at the junction of the thoracic and lumbar spine: You will then increase the curve in your lower back to balance your head over your pelvis decrease the kyphosis in your chest region. The problems created by an unbalanced spine have been previously discussed.

It is becoming increasingly common to see deformity surgery on completely straight spines—with *no* scoliosis or kyphosis. Presumably these surgeries are performed for pain, but there is no medical basis for it. *Do not let anyone perform a major deformity operation on you unless you are significantly off balance.*

Major Surgery plus Major Complication

Early in my practice, I treated Betsy, a woman in her late sixties. She had mild flatback from narrowing discs and had experienced acute low back pain over the preceding six months. Several months of physical therapy had not helped. We elected to do a fusion from T9 to the pelvis and the surgery went perfectly; it only took around six hours, with very little blood loss. My co-surgeon and I felt great about the procedure and we high-fived each other as we exited the operating room.

Making rounds the next morning I was pleased to see Betsy recovering according to the usual post-operative course. A couple of hours later, while I was in clinic, I received a call from her nurse reporting that Betty could not see. Apparently, she hadn't been able to see when I'd visited her, but had thought that it was due to a cloth placed over her face as a routine measure, obstructing her vision. We discovered that during surgery the blood supply to her optic nerves had been interrupted, causing her to go blind. Such interruptions to blood flow sometimes occur in surgery.

I saw Betsy ten years later to remove part of her hardware, which had become too prominent under her skin. She was still blind. In our conversations during that time, I found out that she was now divorced and had been in an unhappy marriage at the time of the initial surgery.

In retrospect, her trunk imbalance was not that bad. Could we have worked harder with her conditioning? Could we have stretched her hip flexors enough to compensate for her flatback and forward bend? Could we have avoided surgery and this devastating complication?

Stable Curves

Some of the most impressive x-rays I have seen were scoliosis films of patients who were over forty. The x-rays revealed curves in their lower backs between 30 and 60 degrees and massive bone spurs on the concave sides of the curves, evidence of the body's effort to resist the progression of the curve. Most of them were seeing me for questions about the deformity and pain wasn't the main issue.

Curve Size

The size of your spinal curve alone, whether it is kyphosis or scoliosis, is rarely a reason to undergo a deformity operation and there is no clear data that identifies curve size as a source of pain. We have already discussed that truncal imbalance is a separate issue from the magnitude of the curves. It is only when the deformity causes other problems besides axial pain that surgery might be a consideration. Other issues include:

- The premature feeling of fullness after eating, or gastric reflux, because the abdominal contents are compressed.

- The bottom of the rib cage rubbing against the rim of the pelvis and causing chronic pain at the point of contact

- The abdominal contents getting pushed into the chest, causing shortness of breath, without interfering with heart or lung function

Summary of Spinal Deformity

The presence of a curve in either a frontal (scoliosis) or side (kyphosis) x-ray of your spine is not in itself a problem. Consider it a structural issue if there is:

- Trunk imbalance
- Instability, as implied by either:
    - Significant progression over a few years, creating corresponding symptoms
    - Collapse of the curve in the upright position compared to lying flat
- Sciatic pain, which, in the presence of deformity, has to be looked at from two viewpoints:
    - The cause of the actual compression
    - The contribution of the deformity
- The size of the deformity is causing abdominal, cardiopulmonary, or functional problems
    - Spinal deformity is non-structural if:
    - The trunk is balanced over the pelvis and is stable
    - The magnitude of curve is irrelevant without other corresponding symptoms
    - Progression of the deformity isn't creating symptoms

6. Compression Fractures

Of the many kinds of spine fractures, the type is determined by

- Direction of the force
- Strength of the bone (age)
- Magnitude of the force

For example, it requires much more force to break the spinal column of someone who is twenty-four, as opposed to that of an eighty-year-old with osteoporosis.

When large forces are directed straight down the spinal column in a young patient, the vertebrae may "explode," sending bone in all directions, creating instability. With less energy applied down the spine, the vertebrae may only collapse down. This is called a *compression fracture* and can occur when a fair amount of force is applied to young bone or minimal force to an older spine.

A compression fracture is usually stable, so by definition it doesn't pose a risk to the spinal cord or nerves. The wall of bone next to the spinal cord is not pushing backwards toward the nerves or spinal cord; instead, the internal vertebral body architecture is compressed, buckling the front wall of the vertebra. It's similar to taking a loaf of bread and squishing it from either end, into a shorter length.

Most fractures occur as a result of a fall. For patients with osteoporosis, it may take only a small force to cause a fracture, and fractures may occur from just the stresses of daily life if the bone is extremely soft. If the fractures occur over enough levels of the spine, a kyphosis will be the outcome. We discussed kyphosis in the previous section; in this section we will limit our discussion to compression fractures of only one or two levels, with a balanced spine.

There are additional conditions, other than osteoporosis, that can cause the vertebral body to spontaneously collapse from minimal forces. Some types of tumors, such as multiple myeloma, leukemia, lymphoma, and metastatic malignant tumors may weaken the bone. Therefore, whenever a compression fracture is detected, your doctor should order a complete workup, including an MRI and blood tests.

Compression Fractures as Sources of Pain

Acute compression fractures are painful. Acute is defined as something that happens suddenly and tissues are injured. The sources of pain from an acute compression fracture are the broken bone and the soft tissues around it, which include muscles, tendons, and ligaments. One exception is a spontaneous compression fracture, which can just "settle" without pain.

When a vertebra fractures, the cortical shell buckles and breaks, stimulating the many pain fibers within the cortical bone. The result is similar to any broken bone in your body: It hurts, and tissues are deformed. It generally takes around 10 - 14 days for the extreme pain to abate; and it doesn't completely disappear until the fracture is entirely healed, usually in 10 - 12 weeks.

The greater the trauma is to a vertebra, the more damage is done to the muscles and ligaments in and around the spine. Because it takes a good deal of energy to fracture a vertebra in a younger patient with strong bones, the soft tissue component of the fracture is proportionally more painful. In older patients, whose bones can break with a good deal less force, the soft tissue pain may be almost zero.

Structural Compression Fracture

Two factors will make a compression fracture the probable origin of back pain:

- Pain is present at the level of the acute fracture within the first twelve weeks of the injury.

- The fracture did not heal.

Acute Fracture

The diagnosis of an acute compression fracture can be made several ways. If a patient has an acute onset of pain and a new fracture is revealed on an x-ray, it is reasonable to consider the fracture the source of the pain. However, there must be a prior x-ray of the area with which to compare it, ideally taken within three months of the new incident.

The current standard of care for a painful fracture seen on x-ray is to obtain an MRI scan, which is more sensitive and specific. MRIs provide valuable information not revealed in x-rays. For example, a special MRI sequence (STIR image) includes a display of blood that, in the case of an acute fracture, would indicate broken spicules of bone. In addition, the MRI scan detects other, more unusual causes of fracture, such as a tumor or infection.

With a positive fracture on an x-ray and excess fluid within the fracture on an MRI, we can be fairly certain that the compression fracture is the source of pain. If the patient is still experiencing pain after three to four months, the fracture may not have healed.

In patients under fifty, the healing potential is so high that this is almost unheard of. But fractures occasionally fail to heal in older patients.

Non-healing Fracture

The diagnosis of a non-healing compression fracture is difficult. To begin with, you need to wait about four months into the healing process before drawing any conclusions. If pain remains after four months, it should be localized to the fractured vertebrae for it to be considered the source of ongoing pain.

If the fracture hasn't healed, the MRI scan will show persistent fluid in the fracture site, and the x-rays may show some progression of collapse in the body of the vertebra. In addition, the bone scan must be positive; that is, it must show evidence that the body is still laying down new bone in its ongoing effort to heal it.

I treated an unusual situation with one patient who was experiencing persistent pain after a compression fracture. Her x-ray was stable, and an MRI showed no collection of fluid. However, the bone scan, which is a measure of healing activity, revealed an interesting feature: The fractured vertebra showed up as a blank spot, indicating that it had completely lost its blood supply. Without a supply of blood, it is impossible for the body to lay down new bone, so the fracture could not heal. The medical term used for this condition is *avascular necrosis* of the vertebral body, and it is definitely a structural problem that must be surgically dealt with. We did solve the problem with a fusion.

Non-structural Compression Fracture (Type II)

In a younger patient (under fifty), it is reasonable to assume the fracture has healed and is stable after four months. If there were ongoing pain, it wouldn't be from the healed fracture; but since there is a fair amount of force required to fracture younger bone, there is significant soft tissue trauma. This would be considered non-structural (Type II) since it cannot be identified on an imaging test. In this case, we would treat it according to the treatment grid in Type IIA or IIB, depending on the state of the patient's nervous system.

If the patient is older than fifty, after three to four month of non-operative care with only minimal improvement, we would order an MRI to check the status of the fracture's healing. If it hasn't healed, the patient would be a Type I problem.

In a patient with severe osteoporosis, if multiple vertebral bodies have spontaneously collapsed, the bone scans and MRIs will be negative. It is hard to determine what allows this to happen. If tests do not reveal an acute fracture, the fracture(s) are not the source of pain providing the spinal alignment remains relatively centered over the pelvis.

Note that this whole discussion about non-structural fractures has been about spines that are balanced. If the fracture causes the spine to decompensate and become imbalanced (such as in severe osteoporosis that causes a forward bend), then the condition needs to be treated as a spinal deformity issue.

Summary of Structural and Non-structural Sources of Pain

The goal of this chapter was to help you, along with the input from your doctor, develop a clear understanding of whether you are in the Type I (Structural) or Type II (Non-structural) category as it pertains to your specific diagnosis. It is the first step of the treatment process and the first job of the surgeon. It is the surgeon's responsibility to determine whether the problem should be surgically addressed, and it is your responsibility to be informed so that you understand each step of the process.

The diagnoses presented in this chapter cover most pain complaints of spine patients. We have discussed what pathology is an identifiable source of pain as opposed to what probably isn't for each diagnosis, with its own defining characteristics. On the surface, this may appear to be too complicated for non-surgeons, but that is not the case. There actually is not that much grey area.

Understanding Spine Surgery

SPINE SURGEONS GENERALLY have one of two objectives when they perform an operation:

1.   To expose and decompress pinched neurological structures;

2.   To stabilize an unstable spinal column.

This appendix describes the procedures surgeons perform on spines to achieve these two principle objectives. The information is divided into three parts:

B.1   The procedures themselves—decompression, fusion, and deformity correction;

B.2   Surgical approaches—how the surgeon accesses the site: from the back, front, or side;

B.3   The magnitude of each procedure.

If you understand the nature of your proposed procedure, you'll be able to carry on a more informed discussion with your surgeon about benefits, the risks, and other possible options.

Review of Spine Neuroanatomy

Spine surgery is technically challenging because your surgeon is performing multiple maneuvers in close proximity to the spinal cord, nerves, and vascular structures. Often the pathology that is compressing the nerves or spinal cord is severe and the anatomy is distorted. Significant force may be required to move muscle and scar tissue. Surgeons are trained to make each move safely, away from the vital structures; but in the midst of thousands of moves a technical complication can occur. The larger and more complex the surgery, the higher are the risks.

The spinal cord starts at the base of the brain in the upper neck and ends at the first lumbar vertebra at the top of the lower back. The cell bodies for the peripheral nerves are located within the cord. The spinal cord is considered part of the central nervous system since it's similar to brain tissue—and extremely delicate; it's more easily injured than the peripheral nerves and does not recover as well after damage or trauma. Any procedure performed in the cervical or thoracic spine carries a higher risk of a severe neurological injury.

As nerves separate from the spinal cord and exit through the openings in the sides of the spinal column (foramina), they are considered peripheral nerves. Some of them are coated with myelin after they leave the spinal canal; this insulation can be compared to rubber coating around a copper wire, which enhances conduction speed. Multiple small nerve roots combine to form larger nerves similar to a cable. The largest nerve in the body, the sciatic nerve, travels down the back of the leg and has contributions from the two lowest levels of the lumbar spine.

Surgery performed in the lower back runs a lower risk of severe neurological damage. Below the first lumbar vertebra there are only peripheral nerve roots, which have exited the spinal cord. These are freely floating in the fluid-filled dural sac. (The Latin term for these rootlets is *cauda equina*, which means "horse's tail.") The presence of so much fluid protecting the nerves within the lumbar dural sac allows the surgeon to retract the dura with less risk to the neurological structures and greater access to anatomy normally hidden by the nerves. In the neck, middle back, and upper back, however, the dural sac cannot be retracted without causing severe neurological damage. Here the spinal cord occupies most of the sac and is more sensitive to pressure and susceptible to damage to its blood supply.

The implication is if neurological injury occurs in the lower back it usually involves only one or, at most, a very few nerve roots. Paraplegia is possible but rare. In stark contrast, if there is damage around the spinal cord, the outcome is usually complete or partial paralysis.

B.1 Spine Surgery Procedures

Spine surgical procedures fall into three general categories:

- Decompression, which relieves pressure on nerves or spinal cord;
- Fusion, to stabilize the spinal column; and
- Deformity correction, to center the head over the hips

Decompression

Several kinds of tissue can impinge on the nerves or spinal cord. Usually an overgrowth of several of these structures combined causes the compression. They are:

- Bone
- Ligaments (tissue that holds vertebrae in alignment)
- Intervertebral discs (the discs that lie between adjacent vertebrae)
- Scar tissue (appearing after any surgery)
- Synovium (thin tissue that lines facet joints)
- Fat

When the problem is located in the central part of the spinal canal, the constriction is similar to the narrow part of an hourglass. The compression is usually circumferential—that is, it surrounds the cord. The goal of surgery is to remove enough of the tissue to restore the diameter of spinal canal or foramen, but not to remove so much as to create an unstable spinal column. The different types of decompression procedures are:

- Laminectomy/laminotomy
- Discectomy/microdiscectomy
- Removal of scar tissue

Changing the shape of the spine with instrumentation and a fusion can indirectly decompress nerves. In some cases, this is the better choice. Some examples include:

- Increasing the height of a collapsed disc with a spacer opens up the foramen and relieves the pressure on the exiting nerve.

- Straightening a bent-forward spine will relieve the pressure on the spinal cord that is draped over the angle created by the kyphosis.

- Correcting a sideways curvature (scoliosis) will open up the foramen on the collapsed side (concavity) and relieve the nerve compression.

Key Surgical Principles of Decompression

Adequate Decompression

The focus of a decompression is to free the spinal cord or affected nerve(s) by removing an adequate amount of bone and/or other constricting tissue. Your surgeon will correlate the surgical findings with the pre-op scans (MRI or CT images) during the procedure; often the surgeon will return to the scans several times to ensure that all impinging material is removed.

Preserving Stability

It is important to remove enough bone to achieve a complete decompression, but not too much. If too much bone is removed, the spine will become destabilized, causing painful excess motion when the patient bends forward or backward. These post-surgical instabilities can be severe.

To prevent instability, it's critical to preserve two structures: the facet joints and the pars (the bone between the facet joints). Your surgeon is aware of these structures, as they are landmarks to finding the nerves. If the patient's bone is strong, more can be removed. Even if the entire lamina is removed, as long as there is enough support on both sides, the spine will remain stable. With soft bone (osteoporosis), the pars may fracture, leaving the spine unstable regardless of the amount of bone left behind.

Patients often wonder how a spinal segment can maintain function even when its entire back is removed. A spinal segment retains its function because most of the forces applied to the spine are transmitted though the vertebrae and discs in *front* of the spine. Even with the back of the dural sac uncovered, the soft tissues, including scar tissue, will not compress the nerves. Stenosis can re-occur at the same level years later from any combination of tissues re-growing into the spinal canal. The types of decompression procedures are:

- Laminectomy or laminotomy

- Discectomy or microdiscectomy

- Removal of scar tissue

Laminotomy and Laminectomy

A laminotomy or laminectomy is performed through an incision in the back of the spine while the patient is face down. The muscles are swept off the bones to expose the back of the spine, revealing:

- Bony lamina (part of the vertebra that protects the back of the spine)

- Facet joints (connectors of the laminae)

- Spinous process (outcroppings of the lamina where muscles, ligaments and tendons attach)

- Interspinous ligaments (connectors of the spinous processes that also resist forward-bending forces)

With any decompression surgery, a bony window is made through the laminae that protect the back of the spine. This allows the surgeon to view any of the above-mentioned "offending" tissues that are compressing nerves and causing your symptoms. When your surgeon has completed the decompression, he or she will be able to clearly see the nerve roots and dural sac, which should at that point be free of any pressure.

Your surgeon may decide to do a laminectomy, which includes the removal of a whole middle section of bone to allow access to the structures in the spinal canal. For example, if the constriction (stenosis) was located between the 4th and 5th lumbar vertebra, the whole spinous process and lamina of L4 would be cut away so that the interspinous ligament between the spinous process of L3-4 and L4-5 could be taken out. Much care is taken to leave enough bone on the sides (pars) so as not create instability. The pars is the strong, border area of bone of the lamina and provides much of the strength to the back part of the spine.

A laminotomy is similar to a laminectomy but with a lesser amount of bony lamina and ligaments removed from one or both sides of the spinous process. The interspinous ligaments and the spinous processes are preserved. Whether your surgeon recommends a laminectomy or laminotomy will depend on his or her preferences and on your specific type of constriction.

Regardless of which procedure is chosen, the surgeon will be looking at the ligamentum flavum, a layer of tissue affixed to the undersurface of the lamina and lying against the dural sac and nerve roots. It must be peeled off and removed in order to view the nerves. This part of the surgery is challenging when the anatomy is distorted. Removing the flavum is a painstaking process, since it's often stuck to the nerves. It's the stage of the procedure where the dural sac may be inadvertently entered, generally not a major problem, but if nerve damage is going to occur, it's usually during this step. Penetrating the dural sac also allows cerebrospinal fluid (CSF) to leak out, so it must be tightly repaired to prevent an ongoing leak. Occasionally the leak is persistent.

Failed Laminotomy, Successful Laminectomy

About six weeks before she came to see me, Rhonda, a middle-aged engineer, had experienced a sudden onset of pain down the side and front of her left leg. She held a high-stress consultant job that required a lot of travel, and she continued to work in spite of rather severe pain. An MRI scan showed a moderate-to-severe stenosis at L2-3, L3-4, and L4-5. There was a superimposed ruptured disc at L2-3, which was clearly the cause of her acute symptoms because it was new, matched her symptoms, and was the most compressed level. As she was anxious to return to work quickly, I elected to perform a laminotomy only at L2-3 on the left side. The surgery went well; she felt better and was back at work within two weeks.

About a month after the operation, Rhonda's symptoms returned. This time the pain ran down the backs of both legs and was severe enough that I immediately ordered another MRI scan. There was still some residual stenosis at L2-3 and the other levels had not changed; they were moderately tight. Although Rhonda was fairly young and active, her discs were flat and her spine was degenerated enough to be stable.

Based on the fact that I had to repeat the surgery within six weeks of the original operation and the spine was stable, I elected to do complete laminectomies at all three levels at L2, L3, and L4. It was important to be able to see the nerves clearly, and I wanted to make sure that I would not have to take her back to surgery a third time. The laminectomies gave me an excellent view of the dural sac and the nerve roots, and I was able to make sure all three levels were completely free. Regardless of a long incision, Rhonda returned to work within three weeks without any leg pain, and her back pain resolved at about six weeks. Years later, she had experienced no further problems.

Laminotomy Instead of Laminectomy

Carolyn came to see me for a second opinion. A 35-year-old woman in great physical shape, she had been injured while performing heavy physical labor and had pain in a classic L5 pattern, starting in her left buttock and running down the side of her upper leg to her calf and her foot.

Carolyn's MRI scan showed a bone spur on the left side at L4-5 pushing on the L5 nerve root. The disc had also slightly pushed backwards, making the compression worse. This was a classic structural problem with an identifiable cause and matching symptoms. There was some mild narrowing at L3-4 but still plenty of insulating fluid around the nerves. She had been counseled to undergo a complete laminectomy at L3-4 and L4-5; but since the corresponding pain down her leg was from L4-5 and L3-4 had minimal pathology, I felt a smaller procedure was more appropriate.

Carolyn's disc spaces were almost normal, and she had no arthritis in her facets that would limit motion. Additionally, she had gained no additional stability from degeneration of the spine. At her age and activity level, it was likely that with a two-level complete laminectomy, she would have significant spine problems over the next ten to fifteen years. The one-level, left-sided L4-5 laminotomy solved her problem.

Discectomy (Microdiscectomy)

As discussed in Appendix A, there are several stages of a disc rupture. First, the disc bulges backwards, causing the ring (annulus) surrounding the center (nucleus) of the disc to begin to give way. As the ring weakens, the bulge increases. If the ring breaks, the nucleus pushes toward the spinal canal. When the nerves are compressed, there is resulting leg or arm pain and/or neurologic deficits, such as weakness, numbness, tingling, or loss of a reflex.

Usually one thin layer of tissue between the herniated disc and the nerves remains. But should the ruptured disc material push through that thin film, it creates a condition called "free fragment." The chemical reaction from the nuclear material touching the nerve root causes a painful, inflammatory response. Each disc rupture has the potential to cause pain from mechanical compression, chemical reaction, or both.

Disc ruptures vary in size from small to massive. Onset of pain is usually rapid and follows the path of the compressed and/or irritated nerve root. A massive rupture increases the chance of neurological deficits, with loss of motor function the most worrisome; but in rare instances there can be loss of bowel and bladder control as well. Compromise of these bodily functions is a true emergency and surgery must be performed immediately. The medical term for this event is *cauda equina syndrome.*

Discectomy, or disc excision, is the operation to remove a ruptured (herniated) disc. It's the same procedure as a laminotomy or laminectomy; except that, once the opening is made in the back of the spine, the surgeon has to look in front of the nerve root to find the offending disc fragment.

Although a discectomy does not compromise the stability of the spine, the rupture leaves a permanent defect in the ring where the nucleus broke through. The ring has no ability to heal itself, and it is not possible to surgically repair the defect; therefore, the disc will never be as strong as it was before it ruptured. A discectomy only removes the pressure against the nerve and does not repair the injured segment back to its pre-injury state. Attention to posture, conditioning, and body mechanics are important to avoid a re-rupture.

Surgical Principles

Similar principles discussed in the laminotomy/laminectomy section apply to the discectomy. The difference is that the problem usually exists in front of the nerve instead of consisting only of pressure on the back of the nerve. Enough bone has to be removed so that the nerve can be viewed and pulled over far enough to excise the disc material underneath.

The procedure is not as straightforward as it might seem. Once the disc has escaped the confines of the ring it can travel in any direction, so it's critical to correlate the pre-op scan with what is seen during surgery. It's common to think that the material has been removed only to find, after further searching, an even larger fragment. Occasionally a significant amount of disc material is left behind ("retained fragment") and an additional operation is needed to remove it.

When searching for these elusive fragments, it's possible to apply too much pressure to the nerve root and cause damage. If the root is already partially damaged, even the smallest amount of additional pressure can make it worse. However, usually the nerve will recover in 12 - 24 months. This is in contrast to the spinal cord, whose recovery is less certain. Reaching under the nerves in the cervical spine is more difficult because of the spinal cord occupies a greater percent of the canal.

The most frequent problem with a discectomy is that more disc material can re-rupture through the same hole, which is impossible to plug. Some disc material must remain within the disc, as it is dangerous to attempt to remove all of it. In the lower back, the aorta or vena cava could be perforated by reaching in too far with grabbing instruments, resulting in fatal bleeding.

Generally, microdiscectomies work well, and patients want to get back to their prior activities without restrictions. However, since your back or neck is not as strong as it was before the rupture, returning to unrestricted activity is risky. Remember, your prior level of activity over time caused the original herniation. With careful adherence to posture and body mechanics that minimizes unsupported bending, the risk can be markedly decreased for the lower back. However, I have seen patients be incredibly careful and still re-rupture. There is not much activity modification that can reduce the chances of a re-rupture in the neck.

The onset of pain with a re-rupture is usually rapid, severe, associated with a specific movement, and in the same distribution as the original rupture. I have seen it happen as early as five days post-operatively and as late as years later. The longest interval I observed was a woman who, while lifting, re-ruptured twenty-five years after her original operation. At surgery, the defect in the ring looked as if it had occurred the day before.

Persistent pain without a pain-free interval after the original operation indicates that there was some disc material left behind (retained fragment), or maybe there was another reason for the pain besides the spine. The gradual re-onset of symptoms can mean almost anything, and the workup has to start from the beginning.

When a re-rupture occurs, the nerve is trapped by scar tissue from the prior surgery and cannot move out of the way as easily. The symptoms tend to be more severe with less chance of resolving. With a first re-rupture in the lower back, most surgeons will repeat the discectomy, which requires dissecting scar tissue instead of working with clean planes. This creates a slightly higher chance of perforating the dural sac and putting too much traction on the nerve; however, most of the time the redo works as well as the first operation. In the neck and thoracic spine, a fusion is usually performed, as it is riskier to free up a scarred nerve root in proximity to the spinal cord. Believe it or not, the disc can rupture again after a re-excision in the lumbar spine. In this situation, most surgeons would do a fusion to prevent another rupture.

Re-Rupture Doing Heavy Work

George was a 33-year-old auto body repairman who'd been in the business since he was a teenager. One day at work his L5-S1 disc ruptured and he had severe pain down the right S1 nerve root distribution, located in the buttock, hamstring, and back of his calf. He also had numbness on the side of his foot and mild weakness in his calf muscles. He had no back pain. His rupture was moderate, and we tried to treat it non-operatively for over eight weeks, including rehab and two cortisone injections, with no relief. He finally elected to undergo a discectomy at L5-S1 through a laminotomy on the right side. The surgery was routine and within a week he was pain-free. George began physical therapy six weeks after his operation. Three months after surgery, he was back to full function and wanted to return to his job.

Returning to fairly heavy work is possible if patients are religious about posture and body mechanics. But unsupported repetitive bending is a major contributing factor to a disc rupture; and with auto-body work, it seemed unlikely that George could avoid it. After several conversations with his employer, we all agreed to let him try.

George did well for six months, until he re-ruptured the same disc at work, with the exact pattern of pain down his leg. Since the re-rupture was smaller this time and his pain moderate, we tried for six weeks to treat him non-surgically; however, he discovered that he could not get back to full function. So, he underwent a re-excision of the disc and quickly became pain-free. But instead of returning to the same job, he was re-trained in a lighter line of work and doing well three years later.

Removal of Scar Tissue

Every operation in the spinal canal leaves scar tissue around the nerve root. When deciding to operate on a patient with a re-rupture, it is often difficult to differentiate disc material from scar tissue. If the surgeon finds a new fragment of disc, the patients do well. But if it's just scar tissue putting pressure on the nerve, the chances of relieving radicular pain are much lower.

Recurrent pain down the leg after nerve decompression surgery is often blamed on scar tissue. But since there is always scar tissue after surgery, I don't find it logical to assume that it's the problem. As discussed in chapter 6, a flare-up of permanent pain circuits is a possible explanation for recurrent pain.

Her Husband—Not a Re-rupture

Laura was a middle-aged professional who had been experiencing pain for over a year. She continued to work, but the persistent sciatica in her left leg was wearing her down. After about three months of treatment, we decided to perform surgery to remove a bone spur and disc material at left L4-5. She did well for over a year; but then her pre-op pain slowly returned. I wasn't convinced that scar tissue on the repeat MRI was enough to be causing her pain.

I sat down with her to find out what else might be going on in her life. She was upset with her husband, a delivery driver, who had rear-ended another car but didn't report it to his employer. When he was found out, he was immediately terminated.

As she worked through the circumstances and calmed herself down, the sciatica resolved.

More About Scar Tissue

To answer the question of whether the scar is causing significant compression, a myelogram followed by a CAT scan provides valuable information. An iodine-based dye is injected into the dural sac; and if the dye flows past the nerve roots without restriction, this indicates the compression isn't severe enough to perform a repeat surgery. If the flow is blocked, I would be willing to consider surgery to remove the scar tissue, hoping that it wouldn't re-form in a way that pinches the nerve. The results in this situation are unpredictable.

With a scar-removal procedure, I worked from the normal anatomy and then approached the distorted scarred-in area from several directions. I wanted to view the whole nerve root and ensure it was completely mobile. If the leg pain later persisted, I wanted to have complete assurance that the nerve had no pressure on it. If so much bone needed to be removed that it de-stabilized the spine, I would combine the decompression with a fusion. This possibility was a part of the pre-op discussion with the patient.

Removal of Scar versus a Fusion

Tom was a 50-year-old ex-carpenter who'd come to me for a second opinion. He'd been disabled with back problems for over fifteen years and had undergone four decompression operations at L5-S1 on the right side. Each decompression had provided him with reasonable relief of his leg pain, but he had persistent low back pain and was on high-dose narcotics. About four months before I saw him, he'd again developed pain down his right leg; it was severe enough that even the high dose narcotics had no effect.

Both the MRI scan and myelogram showed a marked amount of scar tissue compressing the nerve; there was also a hint that the ring around the disc had pushed back slightly, but he clearly had not re-ruptured a disc.

One surgeon had recommended a four-level fusion, and another had recommended a one-level redo decompression and fusion. I agreed that he needed a decompression but I was doubtful about the fusion since his disc was completely collapsed and stable. I felt I could safely remove enough bone to decompress the nerve and not cause instability. After several conversations, we elected to proceed with his fifth decompression operation on that same level. I had reservations about the decision: sometimes the nerves are just damaged and cannot stop emitting pain sensations. The surgery went well, the nerve was completely liberated, and Tom's leg pain decreased by about 80%.

Two years later he was still experiencing his baseline low back pain, but his leg pain was minimal. He maintained his stable dose of narcotics (for the LBP) and was happy with the surgical decision. He would not have had benefitted from an additional fusion, which doesn't solve LBP.

Fourth Surgery with a Fusion

I encountered a similar situation with Mary, 45, one of my colleagues. Over a period of eight years she had undergone three decompression surgeries at L5-S1 for persistent right leg pain. Each of the surgeries relieved her pain and allowed her to quickly return to work. She never experienced significant low back pain.

About one year before I saw her, the same leg pain reappeared. Both the MRI and the CT myelogram scan showed no evidence of another rupture; but there was some ill-defined deviation of the 5th lumbar and first sacral just before they exited the spinal canal.

I wasn't sure what I would find during surgery, based on the scans; and I clearly explained to her that all I could do was to completely un-roof both the L5 and S1 nerves, which required aggressive removal of her bone around the nerves. Since her disc had normal motion, removing this much bone created a potentially unstable spine, so I fused her at that level. We spent extra time under the microscope peeling the scar tissue directly off the nerves. If her pain persisted, I wanted to be sure the nerves were free.

Although I had reservations about going back in for a fourth operation, within two weeks her leg pain resolved and by eight weeks she returned to light work. She was able to perform her full-time job four months post-operatively with no back or leg pain. She was still doing well three years later.

Spinal Fusions

A spine fusion is a procedure intended to bring stability to a part of the spine that is unstable. Instability can result from fractures, tumor, infection, severe degeneration of the facet joints, or from a prior surgery where enough bone was removed to render it unstable. The fusion "welds" the vertebrae together, and the end result is that the segment is now more stable than a normal level.

Fusions make it possible to remove more bone from around the nerves. In some instances, it is the safest option, in that better dissection planes can be defined and visualization improved. However, the fusion creates excess stress above and below it, and there is a significant chance of the spine breaking down over time. So, a fusion is warranted only when a spine is unstable. Pain, in and of itself, is not a reason to perform a spine fusion.

A fusion can be performed across any joint. For example, the ankle may become arthritic from prior trauma or from normal wear and tear. To eliminate painful motion, the joint is surgically destroyed, bone graft material is placed in the defect, and the site is immobilized with hardware. When a bridge of bone forms across the ankle in 3 – 4 months, the patient can put full weight on it. Although the pain is gone, though, the joint is rigid, creating more stress on adjacent working joints in the foot, potentially creating more problems.

Similarly, in the spine, a fusion eliminates movement across a vertebral motion segment by causing a bony bridge to form. The segment consists of two vertebrae, the disc in between, and the two facet joints at the back of the spine. A fusion could span many levels of vertebral segments, the extreme being from the skull to the pelvis. For example, a one-level fusion at L4-5 would include the fourth and fifth lumbar vertebrae, the disc, and the facets between the vertebrae. A two-level fusion from L4 to the sacrum (S1) would include three vertebrae (L4, L5, S1) and two discs (L4-5 and L5-S1).

Obtaining Solid Fusions

Several conditions must be met for new bone to form:

1. An adequate blood supply;

2. Clean, bony surfaces where the grafting material will be in contact with bone;

3. An ample amount of graft material with strong bone formation characteristics; and

4. Little motion across the segment. All of these variables are important.

If even one is missing, the likelihood of a successful fusion is reduced. Placing graft at both the front (anterior) and back (posterior) of the spine, which is often called a "circumferential" fusion, significantly increases the odds of a fusion healing.

Adequate Blood Supply

A healthy blood supply is necessary for delivering cells and proteins that stimulate bone formation. But blood flow is diminished with a history of multiple prior surgeries, because the inevitable scar tissue has less vascular capacity.

Another factor that profoundly affects blood supply is tobacco use. Smoking dramatically decreases the ability of the body to form bone. Most surgeons require their patients to quit smoking before surgery; the longer off cigarettes, the better, although it isn't clear how much time is enough. If a given patient refuses to stop smoking, most surgeons will decline to operate, unless it is an emergency.

Steroids interfere with bone formation and healing, as do the reasons one might be taking steroids, which include kidney disease or failure, dialysis, and any type of autoimmune disorder. All of these factors present obstacles to obtaining a solid fusion.

Bone Graft Contact

During fusion surgery, muscles are meticulously stripped from bones; any soft tissue left between the graft and bony surface blocks healing. Direct contact between the two graft elements is critical. Bony surfaces are roughened up to expose the graft to the bone's blood supply.

Bone Graft Material

Bone formation in a fusion requires placing bone graft material into receptive tissue, which stimulates a response similar to healing a broken bone. Ideal bone graft material has two characteristics: 1) it provides scaffolding for the new bone to cross and 2) it contains proteins that stimulate bone formation (*osteoinductive*).

There are only two osteoinductive graft materials: Your body's own bone (the best source); and a substance called *bone morphogenic protein* (BMP). BMP is equivalent to your own bone in that the protein that stimulates bone formation has been isolated and placed on a carrier material.

BMP is FDA approved for use only in the front of the spine. It can be used in the back, but in such cases, it is considered "off label". In other words, the surgeon has made a decision to perform a procedure that has not been approved by government oversight agencies. There is some controversy regarding the safety of such use, and you should discuss the potential benefits and risks with your surgeon.

Fewer spine surgeons are using the patient's own bone or BMP to obtain a fusion; instead there are numerous "bone graft substitutes." These include cadaver bone that has had some of the calcium removed to expose the proteins that stimulate bone formation (*demineralized bone matrix*); but this is a weak stimulant that is not as effective as your own bone or BMP. There are other carriers that can be combined with a patient's own bone marrow or concentrations of platelets. Some materials are just "scaffolding" that allows bone to cross but does not stimulate the formation of bone. None of these substitutes is as effective as a patient's own bone, and data supporting their use is scarce and confusing.

To justify the use of these materials, surgeons frequently argue that extra pain is associated with harvesting the patient's bone from his or her pelvis. But there are many reasons for continuing to use the patient's own bone. It has the best chance of creating a solid fusion. By creating a small window instead of stripping muscles from the pelvic bones, there is a minimum of graft site pain. A recent paper showed that harvesting your own bone did not cause excessive graft site pain (Lehr). Special bone collection devices also allow the surgeon to capture the small bone fragments that are created during the laminectomy portion of the case. Usually, there is enough bone collected to obviate the need to harvest it from the pelvis.

I encourage you to find out exactly what bone graft material your surgeon is planning on using.

Eliminating Motion

When any fracture in the body is healing, it must be immobilized so that new bone can form. If motion occurs, only scar tissue will form. When spine fusion procedures were in their early years, the only way to stabilize the vertebrae post-surgery was to put the patient in a body cast. The last twenty years, however, have seen major advances in internal fixation devices that minimize motion between the vertebrae.

One advance is placing screws directly into the vertebrae through the pedicle, the tube of bone that connects the back of the spine (laminae) to the vertebral body. These pedicle screws are then linked by rods or plates, which further secures the segment(s).

Depending on how tightly the screws affix to the pedicle and the strength of the patient's bone, these devices will function until the fusion is solid. If a bridge of bone does not form, the construct will fail: The screws will either loosen within the pedicles or the metal breaks from fatigue. This is not as dangerous as it sounds; it just means that there is still motion across the intended fusion segment. It is the bone that creates a rigid fusion, not the hardware.

Placing pedicle screws is now a standard practice because the rigid fixation improves the chances of obtaining a solid fusion. If a fusion doesn't heal, a second operation often has to be performed to repair the weak spot. The use of screws does carry a higher complication rate. The risks associated with pedicle screws deserve further discussion. They include:

- Nerve damage with mal-positioning of screws
- Higher re-operation rate
- Infection
- Breakdown adjacent to the fusion

Nerve Damage with Screw Mal-positioning

Nerve damage is a risk because the screws are large and must be fitted tightly into the pedicle to obtain adequate fixation. Nerves adjoin both sides of the pedicle. Even if just a small thread of the screw pokes through, it might irritate or damage a nerve. In the thoracic or cervical spine, the screw can damage the spinal cord. If the screw is too small, it can pull out before the fusion becomes solid, which is more problematic in patients who have weak bone (osteoporosis). During the operation, steps are taken to minimize the risk of nerve damage from the screw. They are:

- Electrical monitoring of the nerves
- X-ray guidance
- Navigation with 3-D x-rays
- Careful identification of the anatomy and landmarks. With any questions the nerve can be visualized directly by removing some bone.

With these techniques and strategies, returns to the OR to reposition or remove an offending screw have become less common. In spite of everyone's best efforts, though, it still happens.

Higher Re-operation Rate

There is a significant re-operation rate with the use of screws. Depending on the number of levels fused and the strength of the bone, the rate is around 15 - 20% within the few years following the operation (Martin 2007, Pitter). Hardware failure, non-healing of the fusion, and nerve irritation or damage all require returns to the operating room.

Some surgeons feel that hardware should be routinely removed, especially if the patient has significant ongoing low back pain following the initial procedure. But there is no data supporting this as a routine practice. I removed hardware to improve LBP a few times early in my career, but it never resulted in pain improvement.

High-risk Patient Returns to the OR

I performed a one-level fusion on an L3-4 degenerative spondylolisthesis. I had worked with the patient for almost a year on his chronic pain issues and had also waited several months for him to quit his heavy smoking habit. The whole process was almost as much of a struggle for me as it was him; but he was upbeat about his progress and future, and I was excited at his progress. He was 55 years old with heart problems, so we obtained a careful medical clearance that said he could probably tolerate surgery although he was at higher risk for cardiac problems.

He woke up from surgery with most of his pre-operative right leg pain gone; but with a new pain down the front of his left leg. A CT scan showed that the threads of the screw were barely protruding through the bone and touching his 3rd lumbar nerve root. We had a choice of waiting this out, since this type of irritation usually resolves within 6 - 8 weeks. But we elected to go back to the OR, where I made a decision to simply remove the screw, as the fusion would be fine with hardware on only one side. The surgery took only about twenty minutes. About four hours after the operation his heart developed an abnormal rhythm from the anesthesia, which proved fatal for his condition. Both his family and I were devastated. It was a grim reminder of the significant dangers hanging over every surgery.

Infection

Placing pedicle screws prolongs an operation, which increases the chances of infection. A deep wound infection with metal hardware is problematic, since metal has no blood supply to fight it off, and antibiotics alone cannot resolve it. Several return trips to the OR and at least six weeks of antibiotics are required to resolve a deep wound infection with hardware in place.

Breakdown of the Spine Around a Fusion

Every well-executed and solid fusion faces the prospect of a breakdown above and below it. A breakdown can manifest in several ways:

- Spinal stenosis
- Breakdown of facet joints
- Disc rupture or herniation
- Bone spurs
- Fracture
- Deformity

Every level of a normal spine contributes a small of amount of motion when a person bends forward or backward. In a person with young, healthy discs, each segment moves from 10 - 20 degrees. Flexion or extension occurs in a smooth arch with the forces distributed throughout the curve.

Now visualize this arch with one of the segments unable to move. The smooth flow of the motion is altered and there is a "kink" around the stiff segment. This is a concentration of forces not unlike water flowing around a rock in a stream. The effect is even more pronounced when more vertebral segments have been fused. Repeated bending causes damage; however, twisting and impact forces are not a problem.

The chance of breakdown around a one-level fusion is roughly

5% within ten years in the lumbar spine (Frymoyer). It is consistently around 35% when fusing multiple levels in spinal deformity (Kim).

Breakdown can occur quickly, and the problems are severe, including neurological deficits, severe pain, and the spine tilted forwards or sideways. Urgent repeat surgery may be needed. Factors that increase the odds of a breakdown are:

- Patient's age when fusion is performed
- Number of levels fused
- Physical condition
- Frequency of repetitive bending
- Genetics
- Smoking

Although the risk of breakdown can be reduced, it can never be eliminated. During surgery, it is important to leave the ligaments above and below the fusion attached to the adjacent vertebrae. If the surgeon removes the interspinous ligament (which restrains flexion), the increased motion will raise the chance of a breakdown. The problem is made worse if the supporting capsules above or below the fusion are damaged; there would then be few supporting structures to prevent hypermobility at the adjacent segments.

Strict adherence to good posture, body mechanics and conditioning is critical for spine health and preventing further breakdown. Repetitive bending at the waist, especially when combined with poor conditioning, is damaging to your spine *even without a fusion*. Core strengthening takes the load off the spine.

Osteoporosis (fragile, porous bone) greatly increases the chances of breakdown. Any fusion is much stiffer than normal bone, and the contrast to osteoporotic bone is even greater. It is mandatory that your bone density be considered in the pre-operative optimization process.

Spinal Deformity

A spinal deformity operation is major surgery. Few surgeries have higher complication rates and more catastrophic outcomes. For this reason, the decision to undergo such a procedure should be limited to correcting an unbalanced deformity that is interfering with the quality of your life or compromising the function of your heart and lungs. Under those circumstances, the results are rewarding for both surgeon and patient, in spite of the problems. The characteristics that define a deformity as clinically significant are discussed in Chapter 3 and Appendix A.

Principles of Adult Deformity Surgery

The reason to perform a spinal deformity surgery is to correct a deformity. I realize I am stating the obvious, but there is a disturbing trend to perform multiple level fusions on relatively straight and balanced spines. I have to assume the reason is pain. There is little data to support the concept of fusing a balanced deformity for pain and not a shred of evidence that a multiple level fusion is helpful for pain relief in a straight spine.

You might ask, "What is a spinal deformity?" It is a curvature of the spine that exceeds the established norms for that area of the spine. The spine may curve sideways, which is termed, "scoliosis." If it curves forward it is called, "kyphosis." When both forward and sideways curves are present, it is "kyphoscliosis". A spinal deformity is possible in any area of the spine. What is unclear is how many degrees of curvature define an abnormal curve. Most surgeons would agree that curves up to 15 degrees (as measured from lines at each end of the curve) are normal and not a source of pain. However, the point at which a curvature becomes a problem has not been defined.

A major consideration for pursuing deformity surgery is the patient's age. In older adult patients, the deformities are more rigid and the bones often weaker, so it is more difficult to obtain full correction. Medical issues must be more carefully addressed in adults, whose soft tissues are less pliable and more fragile. Blood loss is much higher in adults as opposed to children. Combined with a longer operating time there is a higher chance of a deep wound infection. Younger patients seldom have spurs within the spinal canal; whereas, in adults, there are not only spurs, but also often distortions in the anatomy. Bone is less metabolically active in adults, so it is harder to achieve a solid fusion.

The key issue is whether a "deformity" causes you to noticeably lean forward or sideways. Most people are unhappy with such a posture, although a sideways tilt is better tolerated than pitching forward (Daubs). A decompensated deformity is considered a structural problem when you consider the tilting aspect of it. We can usually straighten the spine, but relieving pain is unpredictable.

The Deformity Operation

Once you take apart the spine in order to straighten it, it has to be stabilized with a multiple-level fusion. A common procedure is a fusion with hardware that extends from the tenth thoracic level down to the pelvis. This spans eight levels and removes all motion across this segment. You cannot bend or twist through the area of your spine that is fused. Activities of daily living such as tying your shoes, personal hygiene and getting in and out of a car are more challenging. Fusions from the neck to the pelvis render your entire spine completely stiff.

The spine in adult deformity is typically rigid, so the first step is to loosen it up at every level that needs correction. If 5 - 10 degrees of correction can be obtained at each level, quite a bit of overall correction is achievable. For more severe and rigid deformities, the spine is cut in two from the back. This is called an osteotomy, and it allows the surgeon to obtain significant correction at the one level. Some spines are unstable enough that they correct just with positioning on the operating table. The general sequence of surgery is as follows:

- Decompressions are performed first. As the shape of the spine will change, it is important to first remove bone spurs compressing the nerves. This will avoid more compression and also aid in loosening the spine.

- For rigid spines, the facet joints are removed in addition to part of the lamina. When a lot of bone is removed to create more motion, it is called an *osteotomy*.

- Screws are placed in the middle of the pedicles and then connected to rods, to create a stable, rigid construct.

- Bone graft material is laid over the raw bone on the back of the spine.

- The rods are bent and manipulated to maximize the correction.

The bone graft will grow under and around the rods, creating a solid piece of bone. With multiple levels fused, there is a higher chance of some areas failing to heal and the rods breaking. It is not dangerous; it just means the fusion is not solid. It requires a detailed discussion with your surgeon whether it is worth the risk to go back and surgically repair these weak areas.

Soft tissue dissection is one of the most important features of a large case. The muscles overlying the spine should be removed from the bone by sharp dissection with the aid of the cautery. The whole muscle mass can be mobilized to each side with minimal trauma. Careful attention to the soft tissues decreases infection risk and blood loss.

B.2 Surgical Approaches

Every spine operation can be performed from one of several approaches:

- Front (anterior)

- Back (posterior)

- Side (lateral)

The approach is determined on the basis of whichever has the highest chance of accomplishing the surgical goal. This is an area where the decisions are mostly up to your surgeon. However, knowing more about these procedures will be helpful if you are considering surgery.

We will center our discussion of surgical approaches on fusions, since they constitute major surgery and require more choices than decompression procedures. During fusions, a combination of approaches is commonly used. For example, placing support and bone graft both in front and back of the spine increases the chances of obtaining a solid fusion.

Placing a Graft in the Front of the Spine

The device used to place bone graft between the vertebrae is called a "cage." A cage is a hollow rectangular or cylindrical device that is filled with bone graft material and placed into the disc space, once most of the disc is removed and the bony endplates of the upper and lower vertebrae are cleaned off. It is critical to create a clean surface area to ensure contact of the graft material with the patient's bone. The cage should be sized and tightly fitted so that it doesn't move or back out.

The cage containing bone graft can be placed into the front of the thoracic and lumbar spine from any of the three approaches; but there is only one possible way to insert the cage into the neck (cervical spine), and that way is through the front.

Cervical Spine

Bone graft between the vertebral bodies in the cervical spine is placed only from the front because the back is blocked by the spinal cord, and the side is impeded by major blood vessels. It is a relatively straightforward approach, as the spine is just below a thin layer of muscle beneath the skin. Caution is required, however: The surgeon must work past the trachea, esophagus and blood vessels that feed the brain. The risks of this procedure include:

- Dysphagia—trouble swallowing for up to six weeks; rarely permanent

- Perforation of the esophagus—serious problem causing an infection that can be fatal

- Displacement of the graft—needs to be surgically replaced

- Stroke—vertebral or carotid arteries to the brain injured

- Death—excessive bleeding or swelling of the soft tissue compressing the airway and cutting off air; can occur 24 – 48 hours after surgery

Thoracic Spine

The cage containing the graft material can be placed in the front of the thoracic spine from either the front, side, or back.

Anterior Approach

The surgeon can approach the spine through the chest, with a procedure called a *thoracotomy*. The operation is performed in the chest cavity with the lungs retracted out of the way, which creates excellent access to the front of the spine. As other surgical techniques have evolved, however, this approach is not used as frequently. It requires a chest tube for a few days after the operation. Risks include:

- Pulmonary problems

  - Lung may not re-inflate, requiring reinsertion of the chest tube

  - Pneumonia

  - Persistent drainage of lymphatic fluid

- Chronic chest wall pain from irritation to the sensory segmental nerves

Lateral Approach

The side of the thoracic spine can be approached with a minimally invasive technique called an XLIF (extreme lateral interbody fusion). It allows access to the spine through the back part of the chest cavity and behind the lungs. XLIF relies heavily on x-rays to place the cage; but the much smaller incision has a lesser chance of creating pulmonary problems. Risks include:

- The tissue surrounding the lung may be entered—not a problem if a chest tube is placed.

- The cage can be placed too close to the spinal cord, causing partial or complete paralysis.

Posterior Approach

Costotransversectomy is a procedure where the approach begins from the back and the surgeon removes the structures on one or both the sides of the spine. Eventually the whole vertebral body in front of the spinal cord is exposed. This approach is usually used when there is a lesion, such as tumor or infection pushing on the spinal cord. The cord can be safely decompressed from the side and front, and the cage can be placed directly in front of the spinal cord. As there is such close, direct access to the spinal cord, this procedure has largely replaced the thoracotomy, even though it is technically challenging. Risks include:

- Lung space can be entered—if not recognized, requires a rapid return to the OR for a chest tube

- The general major complications listed in the first section of Appendix B

Vertebral column resection (VCR) or *posterior subtraction osteotomy (PSO)* are procedures where the spine is essentially cut in two (around the spinal cord), all from the posterior approach. With the VCR, the spine can be moved in any direction. A cage is placed in the front from the back and the whole construct is stabilized with hardware placed into the pedicles. With the PSO, there is no cage placed because a thin bridge of bone is left in the front. The opening created by the wedge of bone removed from the back of the spine is closed and stabilized with hardware. Both the VCR and PSO are considered the riskiest procedures in spinal surgery; but the amount of correction that is obtainable is remarkable, even for rigid deformities. VCRs are usually done in the thoracic spine; PSOs in both thoracic and lumbar spine.

Risks include *all* the dangers of major surgery because of manipulation of the spinal cord, proximity to major blood vessels, high blood loss, and the prolonged time the patient is prone (face down).

Lumbar Spine

In the lumbar spine the ground rules are completely different, since the spinal cord stops at the first lumbar vertebra, which lowers the risk of neurological injury. The dural sac, containing only nerves roots floating in cerebrospinal fluid (CSF), can be retracted well to the side, allowing access to the front of the spine. The approaches and procedure names for placing the cage in front of the lumbar spine are:

- Posterior—from the back, past the dural sac:
  Translaminar interbody fusion (TLIF)

- Lateral—from the side:
  *Extreme lateral interbody fusion (XLIF) or
  direct lateral interbody fusion (DLIF)*

- Directly anterior—through the abdomen:
  Anterior interbody fusion: ALIF

Each of these approaches has its advantages and unique set of complications. Understanding the approach is an important part of surgical decision-making.

Posterior—Translaminar Interbody Fusion (TLIF)

The posterior approach is the one most commonly used for lumbar spine fusions. It allows for excellent decompression; and with bone graft placed in both the front and back of the spine there is an excellent chance of obtaining a solid fusion. The complication rate is relatively low.

During the decompression nearly one-half of a lamina is removed, allowing excellent visualization of the nerves and disc space. After the dural sac is retracted towards the midline, the disc space is prepared for placement of the cage: Most of the disc material is removed and the endplates of the vertebrae are cleaned to allow contact of the cage with bleeding bone. With the bone graft packed into the center of the cage, there is more surface area to allow better healing of the bone. The cage is wedged into the disc space between two vertebral bodies. The rest of the operation entails finishing the decompression of nerves, placing the pedicle screws back to front, and laying more bone graft across the back. Now there is an excellent chance of creating a solid fusion.

Lateral—Extreme Lateral Approach (XLIF/DLIF)

The lateral approach in the lumbar spine is quite different from that in the thoracic spine. The muscles that flex your hips (psoas muscles) originate at the sides of the lumbar spine and largely encase it. This large, thick muscle encompasses the nerves exiting the sides of the spine, making them difficult to see and easy to damage.

In the extreme or direct lateral approach (XLIF, DLIF) a small incision is made through the patient's side over the target disc space. This procedure must be performed under x-ray control and is considered "minimally invasive." Your surgeon must be aware of your abdominal contents, ureters, and great blood vessels; but, unlike the direct anterior approach, these structures are not directly in the surgical field. The nerves that exit the side of your spine *are* directly in the field but can't be seen. So, careful monitoring of nerve function is important throughout the procedure to minimize the risk of nerve damage. The advantage of the XLIF is that you are able to place a much larger cage in the disc space and also correct any collapse. Problems occur because of the size of the psoas muscle, proximity of the bowel and major blood vessels, and our inability to see the exiting nerves. Risks for this procedure include:

- Nerve damage

  - Loss of motor function of a muscle or muscle group— greatest concern is the level of disc between the 4th and 5th lumbar vertebrae.

  - Numbness and tingling down the front of the leg— usually resolves in 2 – 3 months, but occasionally is permanent.

- Bowel perforation—Easily missed and may cause a serious deep infection.

- Perforation of the major blood vessels—aorta or vena cava.

Although there may be some specific advantages to using the lateral approach, using the posterior approach carries less risk.

Anterior—Anterior Interbody Fusion (ALIF)

The anterior approach (ALIF) is usually performed through an incision made in the center of the abdomen. Sometimes it's made to one side or at an oblique angle. The contents of your abdomen, along with the ureters (drainage tubes from your kidneys to your bladder) and great blood vessels to your pelvis and legs (aorta and vena cava) are moved out of the field to provide a clear view of your spine.

The ALIF allows the exposure required for more complex problems such as tumors, fractures, infections, indirect foraminal decompression, and the need to place a large graft. This is less risky for the neurological structures because the approach is in front of them. The large psoas muscle that encases the lumbar spine can be retracted out of the way, allowing excellent visualization of the spinal column anatomy.

The main post-operative issue, even more problematic than incisional pain, is that by manipulating the bowels, they cease to work for 1 - 3 days. The patient becomes distended and uncomfortable. In spite of a low infection rate, the following problems occur more commonly with an ALIF:

- Lymphatic fluid can accumulate in the surgical site. It is painful and requires a drain to be inserted into the site for a week or two. Occasionally, further surgery is needed to solve the problem.

- In patients with compromised arteries from peripheral vascular disease, the blood vessels to the bowel may clot off, cutting off the blood supply. This is a dire emergency, requiring immediate resection of the dead tissues, with a high chance of the patient dying.

- Occasionally, the connective tissues don't heal strongly enough to contain the abdominal contents and a midline abdominal hernia may result. This usually requires further surgery.

- When the patient is a young male, we try to avoid this procedure because of the rare occurrence of retrograde ejaculation, a condition where the ejaculate travels back into the bladder. It generally resolves over the course of a year but may render a person permanently sterile.

- Major organs such as the aorta, vena cava, iliac veins and ureters (tubes connecting the kidneys to the bladder), are at risk for perforation.

Choice of Anterior Approach for an L4-5 Fusion

Susan was an active 50-year-old who had moderate low back pain and severe pain down the side and backs of both legs. The symptoms had come on gradually over the course of eighteen months and were most acute when she stood and walked (she had no pain when sitting). She could relieve her leg pain by bending forward at the waist.

X-rays of Susan's lower back showed an L4-5 degenerative spondylolisthesis and central spinal stenosis. Her L4 had slipped forward on L5 about three millimeters, and the slip increased another four millimeters when she bent forward. (Her disc space height was almost normal.) The MRI scan showed the severe constriction in the middle of her spinal canal. The foramina, where the L4 nerves exited the canal out the sides, were open; often these can also become narrowed. The facet joints at the back of her spine that normally stabilize the spine were eroded and gaped open. With the mobile disc and these joints completely destroyed, the L4-5 level was unstable.

Susan's structural problems (Type I) were severe enough that she required surgical correction before meaningful rehab could be done. She needed a laminectomy to decompress her nerves and a fusion to stabilize this level. As she was so unstable, I chose to perform a circumferential (anterior and posterior) fusion both to provide stability and ensure a solid fusion. I had three choices regarding placing the cage with bone graft in front of her spine.

- TLIF—Susan had a wide disc space that would require a lot of retraction of the nerves to slip the cage past them into the disc. Her disc was at least 15 mm in height.

- XLIF—A good choice except that there is a higher risk of nerve damage at L4-5—especially with a little bit of a slip. The L4 nerve root is located at the dead center of the path of the extreme or direct lateral approach.

- ALIF—There is essentially no risk of damaging nerves and I could place a large cage into the interspace and obtain a precise fit.

I decided to first put the cage with graft into the front of Susan's spine with a direct anterior approach (ALIF), making an incision in the middle of her abdomen from navel to pelvis. The abdominal contents were retracted to the side and we mobilized the large blood vessels (aorta and vena cava), giving us an excellent view of the disc. Indeed, her disc height was an issue and she required an 18 mm cage to tightly fill the gap. I used a single, round threaded cage and filled it with artificial, highly osteoinductive (stimulating bone formation) bone graft (BMP).

We turned Susan over on her stomach do the posterior procedure, which consisted of decompressing the L5 and S1 nerves with an L4-5 laminectomy. We used bone graft from her pelvis and stabilized the level with a pedicle screw construct.

The first two weeks after an anterior/posterior fusion are fairly painful. However, the day after her surgery, Susan's leg pain was gone, and she was able to get out of bed. She left the hospital four days later and started her rehab and conditioning within a few weeks. She reached full function with a solid fusion in about four months. At three-year follow-up she is symptom-free.

Minimally Invasive Spine Surgery

Many spinal procedures can be performed from any direction through small openings with specially designed instruments. The expertise and equipment has risen to a highly sophisticated level. In deciding whether you want an operation performed with this method, there are several important points to consider. (Note that the other common methods we have already discussed are the traditional "open procedures," wherein a larger incision is made.)

I feel strongly that, for any and all procedures, the success of the technical performance depends on the surgeon's comfort level. If a given surgeon does most of his operations with a minimally invasive approach, then he or she will probably do a great job for you. On the flip side, if your surgeon is most comfortable with the open procedure, then he/she will also do a great job. Although I do occasionally perform minimally invasive procedure, I prefer using an open approach. With careful attention to the soft tissue dissection, I've been happy with the results of my procedures. Others perform mostly minimally invasive procedures with excellent outcomes. The point of this discussion is just to illuminate the differences, not to debate the merits of one over the other.

The reason for performing a given procedure should not change because it is being performed through a minimally invasive approach. The anatomical and procedural issues are exactly the same. One of the purported advantages of a minimally invasive approach is that it does not cause "fusion disease." In other words, it results in a lesser degree of trauma for the soft tissues around the spine and therefore less long-term back pain. In my view, "fusion disease" is a problematic term. I will acknowledge that the first two days after surgery are more painful with an open approach. However, the pain is reasonable at discharge in a few days. By the two-week point, the back pain is minimal. Long-term back pain is a rehab issue that I don't feel is affected one way other by the approach.

A fusion is still a fusion whether it's done with a minimally invasive approach or with an open approach. It is sometimes implied that minimally invasive surgery causes fewer follow-up problems, but the same long-term problems of breakdown occur with either one, as there is still a stiff segment created in the middle of a mobile spine.

Almost all the surgical approaches discussed in this chapter can be done with a minimally invasive approach. The exception is a lateral approach at L5-S1.

B.3 Magnitude of the Surgery

The technology that is available in modern spine surgery is remarkable. We are now able to routinely perform procedures that we couldn't even imagine thirty years ago. However, even as we grow in our ability to perform more complex procedures, the indications for surgery and suggested magnitude of the procedure has become increasingly unclear.

This chapter examines the magnitude issue from a complexity perspective. We are concerned with these factors in spine surgery because the risk of complications grows with the complexity of the procedure. Factors that reliably increase complexity and risk are length of the surgery, blood loss, and tissue trauma. Other issues such as smoking, obesity, diabetes, kidney failure, heart problems, lung disease, liver failure, age and general fitness also impact the outcome and decision-making.

The following procedures will be discussed. They are listed in order of increasing complexity and higher complication rates:

- Kyphoplasty/vertebroplasty—Injecting cement into a fractured vertebra though a thick needle. There are some risks.

- Decompressions

  - Microdiscectomy

  - Laminectomy and laminotomy

- Fusions

  - Complexity increases with the number of levels fused

  - Surgery performed through both the front and back of the spine adds risks

  - Osteotomies (see VCR and PSO in Appendix B.2)

Kyphoplasty

A kyphoplasty is a procedure where rapidly-setting cement is injected into a compression fracture to stabilize it, quickly decrease pain and help a patient mobilize quickly. Almost all compression fractures occur in osteoporosis (weak, porous) bone, which makes the procedure more risky.

This is an outpatient procedure typically performed with local anesthetic and IV sedation. It is usually completed within an hour, and the risk of infection is negligible. Semi-liquid cement is injected with a large-bore needle into the broken vertebral body. The cement hardens in 6 - 10 minutes, immediately stabilizing the fracture. Pain relief is often dramatic. Problems occur if the liquid cement leaks back into the spinal canal and hardens against the nerves or spinal cord, causing neurological problems. Rarely it could enter some surrounding veins, travel to the lungs and cause pulmonary compromise. An additional risk can occur when the bone is weak and porous. The needle could penetrate the vertebral body into the abdomen, where cement could compress the great blood vessels (aorta and vena cava).

Decompressions

The choices for decompression surgery are microdiscectomy, laminectomy, and laminotomy.

Microdiscectomy

Most surgeons would agree on microdiscectomy as their procedure of choice to remove a ruptured soft disc in the lumbar spine. It is consistently effective.

The bony anatomy is usually quite normal, and access is straightforward. The goal is simply to remove just enough bone and ligament to reach around the compressed nerve and excise the fragment next to it. Surgeons vary with regard to the use of magnifying loops versus a microscope, type of retractors, etc.; but the basic intervention is the same. Of course, the procedure isn't risk-free: About 10% of patients don't do well for reasons that are unclear, or there is a complication.

One of the worst, but fortunately rarest complications is your surgeon reaching in too deeply with the instrument that grabs the disc material and punctures the aorta or vena cava (both major blood vessels in your abdomen). It is difficult to detect, and the hemorrhaging can lead to death.

Any time you are working around nerves, the sac containing the cerebrospinal fluid can be perforated, creating a leak. Usually the leak can be repaired; but if it continues it increases the chance of a deep wound infection. The infection can spread to the disc, which has a minimal blood supply. It is difficult to clean out the infection without doing a larger clean out that requires a fusion. When the sac is entered there is also a chance of damaging the nerves to the legs, bowel and bladder.

One frustrating complication of a microdiscectomy is performing it at the wrong level. The procedure involves a small incision, and it is easy to be one level off with just a small amount of angle change of the retractor. Occasionally, even a perfectly executed disc excision results in permanent leg pain; the cause is unclear.

Another adverse outcome of a microdiscectomy is that more disc material may re-rupture through the same hole in the ring. There is about a 10 - 15% incidence within 2 years (Carragee, 2006). It isn't possible—or safe—to remove all the material during the first operation.

The majority of painful soft discs resolve without surgery, although waiting it out can be miserable. But if you can endure the pain from the initial disc rupture and completely avoid surgery, there is probably less chance of a re-rupture and scarring around the nerve.

Failed Microdiscectomy

Over 20 years ago, an athletic woman in her forties elected to have her L5-S1 disc removed for sciatica. Since she was thin, the surgery was straightforward and took only about 30 minutes. She did well for about three months; until, during a hike, she re-ruptured more disc material through the same defect at the same level. We tried to wait it out; but the nerve was trapped by scar tissue from the original operation, so it was less likely to heal without surgery. During the second operation I simply removed more disc. That surgery also went smoothly, but she didn't improve. Finally, I performed a "definitive fusion" where I really cleaned out the scar and stabilized it. She continued to have ongoing leg pain, even after trying every treatment and medication possible.

This all occurred well before I knew about the nature of chronic pain, and I'm sorry I didn't have the wide range of non-surgical strategies I do today.

Laminectomy and Laminotomy

There is much debate around the choice of procedures for spinal stenosis. Simple decompression, or decompression combined with a fusion? The treatment of choice is a laminectomy or laminotomy because the addition of a fusion does not significantly improve the outcome (Martin 2019).

Laminectomies and laminotomies are riskier operations than microdiscectomies because the anatomy is always distorted in cases of spinal stenosis. The bones overlying the back of the spine (laminae) are thick, the facet joints are enlarged, and the ligament over the spine is thickened. Often the dural sac that contains the nerves is stuck to these ligaments, so it is more common to tear the dural sac. A torn dural sac can usually be repaired, but sometimes it can continue to leak. Disrupting the dural sac also can damage nerves.

In most cases it is unnecessary to add a fusion. Fusions are performed to provide stability to an unstable spine. With rare exceptions, the spine is stable in the presence of stenosis; in fact, it is more stable than a normal spine, because the facets are enlarged, thus having more surface area to provide support. The discs are usually narrowed and stiffer, which also adds to stability. With careful attention to preserving at least 50% of each facet joint the chances of the procedure creating spinal instability approaches zero.

Some surgeons consistently include a fusion for stenosis because the surgery is "going to de-stabilize" the spine. But a surgeon can preserve enough of the structure to maintain stability, and still take the pressure off the nerves with careful attention to detail. If the spine does eventually become unstable you can salvage it later with a fusion. It doesn't make sense to fuse all lumbar stenosis because there might be an occasional instability. That being said, the incidence of fusions for spinal stenosis has exploded over the last 10 years (Martin 2019).

Many surgeons will recommend a fusion because the patient has back pain in addition to the leg symptoms. We have already established that a fusion is not reliably effective for relieving LBP. By "throwing in" a fusion the complexity of the operation has been significantly increased for little if any benefit.

Adding in a fusion for spinal stenosis creates several problems. First, there is now the unnecessary problem of the spine breaking down around a fusion. Second, where do you stop? In stenosis the entire spine is degenerated. There may be three or four levels that need to be addressed by the laminectomy. Fusing three or four levels is a dramatic undertaking, involving at least six hours of surgery with significant blood loss; versus two or three hours with minimal blood loss. After facing a much greater risk of complications, you will most likely still have back pain.

The overall success rate for stenosis decompressions for spinal stenosis is only around 65% (Herno). One of the reasons for the low success rate, I believe, is that the nerves that are compressed in the foramen are often not adequately decompressed. It is a more difficult area to reach—impossible to access from the inside. Your surgeon should be comfortable with the "extraforaminal approach." It is a simple step to reach the offending bone spur from the outside the spine.

Another reason I attribute to the high failure rate is unrealistic patients' expectations. Many believe that back surgery will relieve back pain, and it simply doesn't.

Fusions

Spondylolisthesis

Both isthmic and structural degenerative spondylolisthesis do well with one-level fusions, and there are pitfalls in not performing one.

The fusion is usually required at only one level, even though there may be several levels of stenosis above and/or below it that are stable. My approach had been to fuse the one level of the spondylolisthesis, and then perform only decompression procedures at the other levels. One case was a 53-year-old woman, on whom I performed a fusion at just one level and decompressed two others. Her leg pain and weakness resolved, and lower back pain dissipated with a full rehab program. Another surgeon had recommended an 8-level fusion from her tenth thoracic vertebra to her pelvis. Currently there is a trend to fuse all levels being decompressed, even though complication rates rise with the number of levels fused.

Complications surrounding fusions have already been discussed. Fusion is a much larger operation than a decompression.

Spinal Deformity

The indications for adult deformity surgery are not well defined. The decision to have surgery largely depends on pain and function. Weak data suggests that deformity surgery might help pain, but it has never been compared to a well-implemented structured spine care program (Kelly). This is especially problematic in light of the complexity of the procedures.

Deformity surgeries are long and incur significant blood loss. The complication rate is over 65%, and often the complications are severe (Pitter). They include:

- Nerve root weakness and/or pain—Nerves pinched or damaged as the shape of the spine is changed, or a screw is mal-positioned

- Paralysis—If blood supply was cut off to the spinal cord

- Blindness—Mostly with prolonged surgeries and greater blood loss

- Massive blood loss—A common occurrence and a reason to stop the procedure

- Pulmonary embolus—A blood clot finding its way to your lungs can cause cardiac arrest and death

- Deep wound infections—Requiring multiple re-surgeries and prolonged IV antibiotics

- Screw mal-placement—Compromising vital structures, requiring return to the OR

- Respiratory failure—From pneumonia or fluid overload, requiring a respirator

- Hardware failure—Pulled out of the bone, often requiring major revision surgery

- Skin breakdown—From muscle flaps and grafting, may require reconstructive surgery

- Spine breakdown—May require major revision surgery for neurological compromise or development of a new deformity.

- Deaths—From complications such as coagulopathies, bowel infarctions, stroke, infection and sepsis, pulmonary embolus, cardiac arrhythmias

This is by no means a complete list. These operations rank amongst the most difficult and dangerous in any field of surgery. In addition to "minor" and "major," I have my own category of complication: "catastrophic." These patients often are returned to the OR many times. There may have been significant vital organ damage. Pain might be worse after surgery. The fallout of a catastrophic set of complications destroys all semblance of a normal life.

Twenty-nine Surgeries in 25 Years

Gordon was a 25-five-year-old steel worker who underwent a discectomy for a ruptured L4-5 disc, an injury he incurred on the job. Although the procedure relieved his leg pain, ongoing low back pain prevented him from returning to work. After two years of physical therapy with few results, he was offered an L4-5 spine fusion. He elected for the surgery, thinking it would solve his lower back pain. That's when the real problems started.

The fusion didn't heal, so after a year Gordon had a third operation to address additional pain. That operation did solidify the fusion but did little to relieve his pain. The following year, a discography revealed that Gordon's L3-4 was a degenerated disc, and he was offered another fusion. The operation was successful this time in fusing his vertebrae; but, again, did not relieve his pain.

Then Gordon's spine broke down around his fusions, creating an unbalanced kyphosis, in which his upper body leaned forward so far that he could hardly see ahead of him. Another operation followed—Gordon's most extensive surgery yet—fusing several vertebrae in his thoracic region.

From this surgery he developed a deep wound infection, which required going back in to remove his hardware, plus several more operations to clean out the area. While these procedures treated the infection, Gordon emerged even more bent over than before, barely able to hold up his head. More surgeries followed to correct this new problem, extending the fusion to the base of his neck.

Infection again followed, and with that, more surgeries to remove the hardware and "re-bend" his spine.

By the time Gordon reached me, he was forty-eight years old, severely bent over, and on high-dose narcotics. He had undergone a total of nineteen operations in eighteen years, never having been able to return to work.

I performed two more operations. The first one was to simply check for infection and remove antibiotic beads that had been left in Gordon's spine. Two weeks later, we went back in and removed four wedges of bone from the back of his fusion, enabling him to stand up straight. Gordon was ecstatic. He could now markedly lower his daily narcotic usage.

However, he was not yet out of the woods. Three months later Gordon developed severe anemia (low red blood cell count) and we discovered bacteria in his blood. We suspected infection in his spine, but the incision looked completely healthy. Even though we kept him on antibiotics for six months, infection returned. After removing the hardware to treat his third major infection, he returned to his bent-over posture. Two more major surgeries followed, to re-straighten him.

With so much hardware in Gordon's spine, it was difficult to keep infection at bay; so, we kept him on low-dose antibiotics. His condition was acerbated by the sheer number of surgeries he underwent, creating dense scar tissue, which has a poor blood supply. He wanted to discontinue the antibiotics, so I sent him to one my colleagues, a specialist who performed a radical surgery to correct Gordon's posture. The goal was to straighten him up enough so the hardware could eventually be removed without him bending back over. But before we could remove the instrumentation, he became infected again.

To date, Gordon has endured around twenty-nine surgeries in twenty-five years. But through all the pain and disappointment, he maintained a heroically optimistic attitude. It is just sad to think that Gordon was robbed of the prime of his life.

Now let's go back and retrace our steps, to see if things could have turned out different. Gordon started out a young, strong steel worker with a ruptured disc and corresponding sciatic symptoms—a Type I scenario with a structural source of pain, and surgery an option. Since I didn't know Gordon then, I can't be sure of the condition of his nervous system; but, being that his was a job-related injury, Gordon was most likely in the IB quadrant of the Treatment Grid, under great stress having to navigate through the Workers' Comp system. Unless his pain was too severe to endure any delay, I would have recommended he undergo a structured rehab program for eight to twelve weeks before surgery.

An appropriate simple decompression was performed at one level, which relieved his leg pain. If I had been the surgeon, I would have explained to Gordon that the surgery was not going to address any back pain he might have. Back pain is non-specific, I would have told him; the source of it is unclear. Thus, I would have managed his expectations and recommended that he continue the rehab program for any lingering back pain.

After his discectomy, when he continued to have low back pain, Gordon entered the IIB group (non-structural source of pain, hyper-vigilant nervous system). Several of his chart notes, mentioning how angry he was, bear this out. More surgery is not an option for a Type II condition.

Being young and motivated, Gordon had a good chance of solving his back pain and returning to a normal life. Every one of the surgeries that followed was a direct result of the one lumbar 4-5 level fusion and the spine breaking down around it. It was an unnecessary, ineffective operation that defined the rest of Gordon's life.

Gordon's case is not unusual, except for the sheer number of surgeries he endured. It is common for a first operation to release a cascade of problems that would otherwise have not occurred. I saw variations on this theme every week of my professional life, many with even worse outcomes.

ACKNOWLEDGMENTS

THIS BOOK WAS MADE POSSIBLE BY many people that I would like to deeply thank. My wife, Babs, tolerated many hours on her own while I spent time writing the manuscript. She also is responsible for publishing it along with the rest of my team, Mark Mendonca and Tom Masters. Ray Bunnage is a good friend, who developed an unusual hobby of deeply understanding current neuroscience research and has taught me much.

Marilyn Alan is a remarkable content and copy editor. She is responsible for creating a concise presentation of these ideas. The book cover was designed by James Rothbart.

Mark Owens, PhD, and Sachit Eagan were kind enough to share their near misses with unnecessary spine surgery in the Foreword.

Joel Konikow, MD; Ray Bunnage; Stuart Eivers, DPT; and Robin Shapiro took time to read the manuscript in detail and make timely recommendations.

My practice team members, consisting of Angela Heilbrunn, RN; Sarah Jane Spencer, PA-C; Terry Hudson, MA; Sheryl Schindler, PCC; Cara Cook, ARNP; Katie Rupe, RN; and Andrea Pertoso, PA-C were remarkably committed to individually delivering the highest quality of care for every patient. It was through all our efforts that we gradually learned how to make better decisions and best prepare patients for surgery. Our non-operative care evolved to the point that many patients with surgical problems cancelled surgery because their pain had resolved.

GLOSSARY

Acute—Sudden onset, severe; requiring immediate attention.

Adrenaline—A "fight or flight" hormone secreted by the adrenal glands in response to a real or perceived threat. Effects include increased heart rate, sweating, rapid breathing, muscle tension, and agitation.

Annulus—The multi-layer ring of tissue of the intervertebral disc that surrounds and contains the semi-gelatinous nucleus. The annulus contains many pain receptors, as opposed to the nucleus, which contains none.

Anterior—Toward the front of the body. For example, the vertebral body is anterior to (in front of) the spine.

Anxiety—Unpleasant feeling generated by elevated stress hormones such as adrenaline, cortisol and histamines.

Arthritis—Erosion of the smooth, hyaline cartilage found on many joint surfaces. The cartilage provides a lubricated, water-rich layer to allow sustained painless motion. Erosion can occur from wear and tear, trauma and inflammation. The only true cartilaginous joints in the spine are located in the facet joint on the back of the spine. Neither they nor arthritis in the front of the spine been proven to be consistent sources of pain.

Axial—With reference to the center of the body, as opposed to the arms and legs.

Bulging disc—A condition resulting from the ring around the center of the disc breaking down, allowing nuclear material to be bulge out.

Cauda equina—Latin for "horse's tail," small peripheral nerve roots afloat in cerebral spinal fluid at the level below the first lumbar vertebra, where the spinal cord ends .

Cauda equina Syndrome—Sudden onset of leg numbness and weakness and loss of bladder and bowel function from compression of nerves in the lumbar spine, below the tip of the spinal cord.

Central nervous system—The brain and spinal cord.

Cerebrospinal fluid (CSF)—Clear fluid contained in the dural sac that bathes and nourishes the neural structures within the skull and spinal canal.

Chondromalacia patella—Pain under the kneecap associated with softening of the cartilage between the patella and end of the femur. It is especially sensitive when going up and down stairs.

Chronic—Long-term, persistent condition.

Chronic pain—An indelible memory embedded in the nervous system that continually accumulates associations with an ever-increasing number of life experiences. Also defined as pain lasting more than three months.

Claudication—Sensation of diffuse heaviness, weakness and fatigue in the legs caused by walking and/or standing. May be caused by compression of the nerves of the cauda equina below the spinal cord, or the lack of blood supply, caused by peripheral vascular disease.

Compression fracture—A fracture of the vertebral body resulting from force being applied directly in line with the spinal column (axial loading).

Congenital spinal stenosis—Spinal canal that has a smaller diameter than normal.

Cortisol—Stress hormone that regulates metabolism and the immune system. One of two hormones (the other being Adrenaline) considered most responsible for preparing the body to fend off internal and external threats to survival.

Degenerative disc disease—Not an actual disease; the disc's normal process of losing water content and flexibility as the body ages. A more accurate term is "normally aging disc."

Disc—Hydraulic structure that provides both flexibility and support between two vertebrae, consisting of a ring and a nucleus made of semi-gelatinous material. Also called "Intervertebral disc."

Discogram—A procedure to identify a disc responsible for back pain that has been demonstrated to be unreliable. An iodine dye is injected into a lumbar disc in an attempt to reproduce the patient's "usual" low back pain. It is considered positive if the patient's usual back pain is reproduced.

DOC—Acronym for "Direct your Own Care." A structured rehabilitation program based on documented effective medical treatments that address all relevant aspects of chronic pain. The process is largely self-directed.

Dural sac—A layer of connective tissue that encompasses the brain, spinal cord and cauda equina. It is filled with cerebrospinal fluid, which provides nutrition and protection.

Expressive writing—Writing down positive or negative thoughts and feelings on paper and immediately destroying them. The intention is to detach from one's thoughts.

Facets—Two small joints in the back of each level of the spine, with the same structure as all other articular joints (including cartilage and containment by a capsule of connective tissue).

Failed back surgery syndrome (FBSS)—Collection of symptoms attributed to patients who have undergone multiple failed back surgeries.

Flatback—Decreased lordosis (reverse curvature) in the lumbar spine, occasionally resulting in a tilted forward posture that requires bend the knees to stand up straight.

Foramina/Foramen/Foraminal—Small openings at each level of the spinal column that contain the exiting nerves.

Functional MRI (fMRI)—An imaging study that can record brain activity associated with specific activities and emotions, by injecting a labeled glucose. (Glucose is the brain's energy source.)

Fusion—Creation of a solid bridge of bone across a joint to prevent motion.

Herniated disc—A condition where the semi-liquid vertebral nucleus breaks through the peripheral ring (annulus). Also called "ruptured" disc.

Iliotibial (IT) band—A wide band of tendon that originates at the pelvis, reaches to the side of the knee, and stabilizes the trunk during walking.

Instability/Unstable—When any structure of the body that is intended to provide support in any direction fails to do so.

Intervertebral disc—Hydraulic structure that provides both flexibility and support between two vertebrae, consisting of a ring and a nucleus made of semi-gelatinous material. Also called "disc."

Kyphosis—forward curvature of the spine, the opposite of lordosis.

Lamina—Layer of bone covering the back of the spinal canal; connected to the vertebral body by the pedicle.

Laminectomy—Surgical removal of the central part of the bony lamina that protects the back part of the spinal elements. The surgical goal is to remove pressure on neural elements.

Laminotomy—a smaller version of a laminectomy. Smaller openings are made on one or both sides of the spinous process, allowing more bone to be left intact. The neural elements are still relieved of pressure.

Lateral—Refers to the side of the body.

Lordosis—Backwards curvature of the spine both in the neck and lower back. Opposite of kyphosis.

Microdiscectomy—Surgical procedure to remove a ruptured (herniated) disc, using a microscope for lighting and magnification.

Myelin—Fatty substance that surrounds nerve cells and speeds conduction of impulses; similar the insulation around an electric wire.

Myelopathy—Neurological symptoms created by spinal cord compression. Symptoms are diffuse and include clumsiness, poor dexterity, loss of balance, spastic bladder, diffuse numbness, tingling, and weakness.

Neurological—Anything to do with the nervous system.

Neuroplasticity—The brain's capacity to physically adapt and change at any age.

Nociception—Nervous system's response to harmful sensory input, stimulating physiological and neuromuscular activity to keep you safe. Pain is one of the warning signals.

Non-structural pain—Pain that arises from soft tissues or produced by the nervous system, without an identifiable anatomical abnormality.

Nucleus—Gelatinous material residing inside the vertebral bodies and contained by a ring of tissue called the "annulus."

Pain generator—An identifiable source of pain. Insofar as the concept defines pain as an "input," however, it is flawed; all pain is an output generated by the brain.

Pedicle—Hollow cylinder of bone connecting the lamina in the back to the vertebral body in the front of the spine. Nerves pass directly under the pedicles.

Pedicle screw—Metal alloy screw placed through the pedicle into the vertebral body that provides anchor points into the spine for insertion of rods or plates to stabilize the spinal column.

Peripheral nervous system—Any nerves that are not part of the brain or spinal cord, including motor and sensory nerves, cranial nerves and the autonomic nervous system. PNS transmits input from the environment to the central nervous system.

Physiology—The functions of living organisms.

Posterior—The back of a structure; i.e. the lamina is posterior to (in back of) the spinal canal and vertebral body.

Prehab—Organized rehabilitation program employed to prepare for undergoing a procedure. The Direct your Own Care (DOC) process is one example.

Proprioception—Awareness of your body's movement and position in space.

Pseudarthrosis—Failure of a bony bridge to form, resulting in the formation of scar tissue, which doesn't provide the intended rigidity or stability.

Radiculopathy—Pain that travels down the arm or leg along the path of a nerve root. This pain pattern requires caution in determining the cause, because it specifically points to a spinal source.

Reprogramming—Creating alternate neural pathways to replace learned responses to stimuli.

Ruptured disc—A condition where the semi-liquid vertebral nucleus breaks through the peripheral ring (annulus). Also called "herniated disc."

Scoliosis—Sideways curvature of the spine.

Segmental collapse—Narrowing of one side of a vertebral segment, causing a concavity in the spinal alignment and possibly trapping the exiting nerve.

Spinal column—Sum total of the supporting structures making up the spine from the base of the skull to the pelvis.

Spinal cord—Contained in the spinal canal, the extension of brain tissue to the upper lumbar spine.

Spinal decompression—Procedures or interventions that relieve pressure on neural structures.

Spine fusion—Creation of a solid bridge of bone across a joint, to prevent motion.

Stable/Stability—Firmness of position provided by a supporting structure.

Vertebral body—Cylindrical, bony part of the front of the spinal column that provides most of the spine's support.

Vertebral segment/Motion segment—Unit of the spine composed of a vertebra–disc–vertebra combination.

REFERENCES

Foreword

Baikie, KA and K Wilhelm. "Emotional and physical health benefits of expressive writing." *APT* (2005); 11: 338 - 346.

Boden, SD et al. "Abnormal magnetic-resonance scans of the lumbar spine in asymptomatic subjects: A prospective investigation." *Journal of Bone and Joint Surgery* (1990); 72: 403 - 8.

Carragee, EJ et al. "A Gold Standard Evaluation of the 'Discogenic Pain' Diagnosis as Determined by Provocative Discography." *Spine* (2006) 31: 2115 - 2123.

Chen, X et al. "Stress enhances muscle nociceptor activity in the rat." *Neuroscience* (2011); 185: 166 - 173.

Franklin, GM et al. "Outcome of lumbar fusion in Washington State Workers' Compensation." *Spine* (1994); 19: 1897 - 1903.

Hanscom, D. *Back in control: A surgeon's roadmap out of chronic pain* (2nd edition). Seattle, WA: Vertus Press, 2016.

Hashmi, JA et al. "Shape shifting pain: Chronification of back pain shifts brain representation from nociceptive to emotional circuits." *Brain* (2013); 136: 2751 - 2768.

Owens, M and D Owens. *The Cry of the Kalahari.* New York: Houghton Mifflin Harcourt Publishing Company, 1984.

Perkins, FM and H Kehlet. "Chronic pain as an outcome of surgery: A Review of Predictive Factors." *Anesthesiology* (2000); 93: 1123 - 1133.

Introduction

Franklin, GM et al. "Outcome of lumbar fusion in Washington State Workers' Compensation." *Spine* (1994); 19: 1897 - 1903.

Hanscom, D. *Back in Control: A Spine Surgeon's Roadmap Out of Chronic Pain.* Seattle, WA: Vertus Press, 2012.

Hanscom, D. *Back in control: A surgeon's roadmap out of chronic pain* (2nd edition). Seattle, WA: Vertus Press, 2016.

Schubiner, H with M Betzold, M. *Unlearn Your Pain: A 28-Day Process to Reprogram Your Brain* (2nd edition). Pleasant Ridge, MI: Mind Body Publishing, 2016.

Chapter 1

Eisenberger, N. "The neural bases of social pain: Evidence for shared representations with physical pain." *Psychosomatic Medicine* (2012); 74: 126 - 135.

Hashmi, JA et al. "Shape shifting pain: Chronification of back pain shifts brain representation from nociceptive to emotional circuits." *Brain* (2013); 136: 2751 - 2768.

Song, H et al. "Association of stress-related disorders with subsequent autoimmune disease." *Journal of the American Medical Association* (2018); 319: 2388 - 2400.

Chapter 2

Boden, SD et al. "Abnormal magnetic-resonance scans of the lumbar spine in asymptomatic subjects: A prospective investigation." *Journal of Bone and Joint Surgery* (1990); 72: 403 - 8.

Carragee, EJ et al. "A Gold Standard Evaluation of the 'Discogenic Pain' Diagnosis as Determined by Provocative Discography." *Spine* (2006) 31: 2115 - 2123.

Edwards, RR et al. "Pain, catastrophizing, and depression in the rheumatic diseases." *Nature Reviews Rheumatology* (2011); 7(4): 216 - 224.

Perkins, FM and H Kehlet. "Chronic pain as an outcome of surgery: A Review of Predictive Factors." *Anesthesiology* (2000); 93: 1123 - 1133.

Chapter 3

Abbass, A. "Somatization: diagnosing it sooner through emotion-focused interviewing." *Journal of Family Practice* (2005); 54: 215 - 24.

Chen, X et al. "Stress enhances muscle nociceptor activity in the rat." *Neuroscience* (2011); 185: 166 - 173.

Giesecke, T et al. "Evidence of augmented central pain processing in idiopathic chronic low back pain." *Arthritis and Rheumatism* (2004); 50: 613 - 623.

Hashmi, JA et al. "Shape shifting pain: Chronification of back pain shifts brain representation from nociceptive to emotional circuits." *Brain* (2013); 136: 2751 - 2768.

Mansour, AR et al. "Chronic pain: The role of learning and brain plasticity." *Restorative Neurology and Neuroscience* (2014); 32: 129 - 139.

Nachemson, A. "Advances in low back pain." *Clinical Orthopedics and Clinical Research* (1985); 200: 266 - 278.

Schubiner, H. with M. Betzold, M. *Unlearn Your Pain: A 28-Day Process to Reprogram Your Brain* (2nd edition). Pleasant Ridge, MI: Mind Body Publishing, 2016.

Weddell, G and J. Harpman. "The neurohistological basis for the sensation of pain provoked from deep fascia, tendon, and periosteum." *Journal of Neurology and Psychiatry* (1940); 3(4): 319 - 328.

Chapter 4

Abbass, A, D Lovas and A Purdy. "Direct diagnosis and management of emotional factors in chronic headache patients." *Cephalagia* (2008); 28: 1305 - 1314.

Agmon, M and G Armon. "Increased insomnia symptoms predict the onset of back pain among employed adults." PLoS ONE (2014); 9(8): e103591. doi: 10.1371/journal.pone.0103591.

Anda, RF et al. "The enduring effects of abuse and related adverse experiences in childhood: A convergence of evidence from neurobiology and epidemiology." *European Archives of Psychiatry and Clinical Neuroscience* (2006); 256: 174 - 186.

Chen, X et al. "Stress enhances muscle nociceptor activity in the rat." *Neuroscience* (2011); 185: 166 - 173.

Cigna U.S. Loneliness Index: Survey of 20,000 Americans Examining Behaviors Driving Loneliness in the United States. (2018); 1 - 61.

Davis, DA et al. "Are reports of childhood abuse related to the experience of chronic pain in adulthood? A Meta-analytic Review of the Literature." *Clinical Journal of Pain* (2005); 21: 398 - 405.

Dube, SR et al. "Cumulative childhood stress and autoimmune diseases in adults." *Psychosomatic medicine* (2009); 71: 243 - 250.

Eisenberger N. "The neural bases of social pain: Evidence for shared representations with physical pain." *Psychosomatic Medicine* (2012); 74: 126 - 135.

Fredheim OM et al. "Chronic non-malignant pain patients report as poor health-related quality of life as palliative cancer patients." *Acta Anaesthesiologica Scandinavica* (2008); 52: 143 - 148.

Hawkley, LC and J Cacioppo. "Loneliness matters: A theoretical and empirical review of consequences and mechanisms." *Annals of Behavioral Medicine* (2010); 40: 1 - 14.

Institute of Medicine (IOM) Report. *Relieving pain in America: a blueprint for transforming prevention, care, education, and research.* Washington, DC: National Academies Press, 2011.

Karaman, S et al. "Prevalence of sleep disturbance in chronic pain." *European Review for Medical and Pharmacological Sciences* (2014); 18: 2475 - 2481.

Linton, SJ. "A review of psychological risk factors in back and neck pain." *Spine* (2000); 25: 1148 - 1156.

O'Connor, AB. "Neuropathic pain: Quality-of-life impact, costs and cost effectiveness of therapy." *Pharmacoeconomics* (2009); 27(2): 95 - 112.

Perkins, FM and H Kehlet. "Chronic pain as an outcome of surgery: A Review of Predictive Factors." *Anesthesiology* (2000); 93: 1123 - 1133.

Rahe, R et al. "Social stress and illness onset." *Journal of Psychosomatic Research* (1964); 8: 35.

Sarno, JE. *Healing Back Pain: The Mind-Body Connection.* New York: Warner Books, 1991.

Schubiner, H. with M. Betzold, M. *Unlearn Your Pain: A 28-Day Process to Reprogram Your Brain* (2nd edition). Pleasant Ridge, MI: Mind Body Publishing, 2016.

Schug, SA and EM Pogatzki-Zahn. "Chronic pain after surgery or injury." *Pain: Clinical Updates. International Association for the Study of Pain* (2011); 19: 1 - 5.

Seminowicz DA, et al. "Effective treatment of chronic low back pain in humans reverses abnormal brain anatomy and function." *The Journal of Neuroscience* (2011); 31: 7540 - 7550.

Song, H et al. "Association of stress-related disorders with subsequent autoimmune disease." *Journal of the American Medical Association* (2018); 319: 2388 - 2400.

Torrance, N et al. "Severe chronic pain is associated with increased 10-year mortality: A cohort record linkage study. *European Journal of Pain* (2010); 14: 380 - 386.

Chapter 5

Brox, JI, et al. "Randomized clinical trial of lumbar instrumented fusion and cognitive intervention and exercises in patients with chronic low back pain and disc degeneration." *Spine* (2003); 28(17): 1913 - 1921.

Chen, X et al. "Stress enhances muscle nociceptor activity in the rat." *Neuroscience* (2011); 185: 166 - 173.

Fairbanks, J et al. "Randomized controlled trial to compare surgical stabilization of the lumbar spine with an intensive rehabilitation program for patients with chronic low back pain: the MRC spine stabilization trial." *BMJ* (2005); doi:L10:10.1136/bmj.38441.BF.

Franklin, GM et al. "Outcome of lumbar fusion in Washington State Workers' Compensation." *Spine* (1994); 19: 1897 - 1903.

Fritzell, P et al. "Swedish Lumbar Spine Study Group: Lumbar fusion versus non-surgical treatment for LBP." *Spine* (2001); 26: 2521 - 2532.

Hanscom, D. *Back in control: A surgeon's roadmap out of chronic pain* (2nd edition). Seattle, WA: Vertus Press, 2016.

Kim, JK et al. "Proximal junctional kyphosis in adult spinal deformity after segmental posterior spinal instrumentation and fusion." *Spine* (2008); 33: 2179 - 2184.

Lieberman, SM et al. "Reducing the growth of Medicare spending: geographic versus patient-based strategies." *Health Affairs* (2003); DOI 10.1377/hlthaff.W3.603 ©2003 Project HOPE.

Nguyen, TH et al. "Long-term outcomes of lumbar fusion among worker's compensation subjects." *Spine* (2010); 20: 1 - 11.

Perkins, FM and H Kehlet. "Chronic pain as an outcome of surgery: A Review of Predictive Factors." *Anesthesiology* (2000); 93: 1123 - 1133.

Chapter 6

Agmon, M and G Armon. "Increased insomnia symptoms predict the onset of back pain among employed adults." PLoS ONE (2014); 9(8): e103591. doi: 10.1371/journal.pone.0103591.

Barrett, LF. *How emotions are made.* New York: Houghton Mifflin Harcourt Publishing, 2018.

Brand, P and P Yancey. *Pain: The gift nobody wants.* New York: Harper Collins, 1993.

Chen, X et al. "Stress enhances muscle nociceptor activity in the rat." *Neuroscience* (2011); 185: 166 - 173.

Eisenberger N. "The neural bases of social pain: Evidence for shared representations with physical pain." *Psychosomatic Medicine* (2012); 74: 126 - 135.

Gallagher, P et al. "Phantom limb pain and RLP." *Disability and Rehabilitation* (2001); 23: 522 - 530.

Giesecke, T et al. "Evidence of augmented central pain processing in idiopathic chronic low back pain." *Arthritis and Rheumatism* (2004); 50: 613 - 623.

Fredheim OM et al. "Chronic non-malignant pain patients report as poor health-related quality of life as palliative cancer patients." *Acta Anaesthesiologica Scandinavica* (2008); 52: 143 - 148.

Harari, YN. *Sapiens: A Brief History of Humankind.* New York: Harper, 2015.

Hashmi, JA et al. "Shape shifting pain: Chronification of back pain shifts brain representation from nociceptive to emotional circuits." *Brain* (2013); 136: 2751 - 2768.

Karaman, S et al. "Prevalence of sleep disturbance in chronic pain." *European Review for Medical and Pharmacological Sciences* (2014); 18: 2475 - 2481.

Lent, R et al. "How many neurons do you have? Some dogma of quantitative neuroscience under revision." *European Journal of Neuroscience* (2012); 35: 1 - 9.

Mansour, AR et al. "Chronic pain: The role of learning and brain plasticity." *Restorative Neurology and Neuroscience* (2014); 32: 129 - 139.

Moseley, L and A Arntz. "The context of a noxious stimulus affects the pain it evokes." *Pain* (2007); 133: 64 - 71.

O'Connor, AB. "Neuropathic pain: Quality-of-life impact, costs and cost effectiveness of therapy." *Pharmacoeconomics* (2009); 27(2): 95 - 112.

Ohayon, MM. "Relationship between chronic painful physical condition and insomnia." *Jourrnal of Psychiatric Research* (2005); 39: 151 - 159. Doi:10..1016/j.jpsychires.2004.07.001.

Onen, SH, et al. "The effects of total sleep deprivation, selective sleep interruption and sleep recovery on pain tolerance thresholds in healthy subjects." *Journal of Sleep Research* (2001); 10: 35 - 42.

Sarno, John. *Mind Over Back Pain: A Radically New Approach to the Diagnosis and Treatment of Back Pain.* Berkley, CA: Berkeley, 1999.

Torrance, N et al. "Severe chronic pain is associated with increased 10-year mortality: A cohort record linkage study." *European Journal of Pain* (2010); 14: 380 - 386.

Trincker, D. (German physiologist). Lecture at University of Kiel on the 300-Year Anniversary of the founding of the University of Kiel, 1965.

Wegener, DM et al. "Paradoxical effects of thought suppression. *Journal of Personality and Social Psychology* (1987); 53: 5 - 13.

Chapter 7

Agmon, M and G Armon. "Increased insomnia symptoms predict the onset of back pain

among employed adults." PLoS ONE (2014); 9(8): e103591. doi: 10.1371/journal.pone.0103591.

Apkarian, AV et al. "Chronic back pain is associated with decreased prefrontal and thalamic gray matter density." *Journal of Neuroscience* (2004); 24: 10410 - 10415.

Asmundson, GJG and J Katz. "Understanding the co-occurrence of anxiety disorders and chronic pain: State-of-the-art." *Depression and Anxiety* (2009); 26: 888 - 901.

Bigos, SJ et al. "A Prospective Study of Work Perceptions and Psychosocial Factors Affecting the Report of Back Injury." *Spine* (1991); 16: 1 - 16.

Brown, S and C Vaughan. *Play: How it Shapes the Brain, Opens the Imagination, and Invigorates the Soul.* New York: Penguin, 2010.

Craufurd, DIO et al. "Life events and psychological disturbances in patients with low back pain." *Spine* (1990); 15(6): 490 - 4.

Deyo, RA. "Lumbar degenerative disc disease: Still more questions than answers." *The Spine Journal* (2015); 15: 272 - 274.

Dragananski et al. "Temporal and spatial dynamics of brain structure changes during extensive learning." *The Journal of Neuroscience* (2006); 26: 6314 - 6317.

Eisenberger, N et al. "Does rejection hurt? An fMRI study of social exclusion." *Science* (2003); 290.

Dworkin, RH et al. "Unraveling the effects of compensation, litigation, and employment on treatment response in chronic pain." *Pain* (1985); 23: 4959.

Edwards, RR et al. "Pain, catastrophizing, and depression in the rheumatic diseases." *Nature Reviews Rheumatology* (2011); 7(4): 216 - 224.

Felitti, VJ et al. "The relationship of adult health status to childhood abuse and household dysfunction." *American Journal of Preventive Medicine* (1998); 14: 245 - 258.

Greenwood, KA et al. "Anger and persistent pain: Current status and future directions." *Pain* (2003); 103: 1–5.

Gibbs, J et al. "Preoperative serum albumin level as a predictor of operative mortality and morbidity." *The Archives of Surgery* (1990); 134: 36 - 42.

Halpin, RJ et al. "Standardizing care for high-risk patients in spine surgery." *Spine* (2010); 25: 2232 - 2238.

Hanscom, D. *Back in control: A surgeon's roadmap out of chronic pain* (2nd edition). Seattle, WA: Vertus Press, 2016.

Institute of Medicine. Relieving *Pain in America: A blueprint for transforming prevention, care, education, and research.* Washington, DC: National Academies Press, 2011.

Kerezoudis, P et al. "Returns to the operating room after neurosurgical procedures in a tertiary care academic medical center: Implications for health care policy and quality improvement." *Neurosurgery* (2018); 0: 1 - 10.

Song, H et al. "Association of stress-related disorders with subsequent autoimmune disease." *Journal of the American Medical Association* (2018); 319: 2388 - 2400.

Stung, JP. "The chronic disability syndrome." In Aronoff, GM (ed). *Evaluation and Treatment of Chronic Pain.* Baltimore, MD: Urban & Schwarzenberg, 1985.

Torrance, N et al. "Severe chronic pain is associated with increased 10-year mortality: A cohort record linkage study. *European Journal of Pain* (2010); 14: 380 - 386.

Trincker, D. (German physiologist). Lecture at University of Kiel on the 300-Year Anniversary of the founding of the University of Kiel, 1965.

Young, AK et al. "Assessment of presurgical psychological screening in patients undergoing spine surgery." *Journal of Spinal Disorders and Techniques* (2014); 27: 76 - 79.

Chapter 8

Best, N et al. "Outpatient lumbar decompression in 233 patients 65 years of age or older." *Spine* (2007); 32: 1135 - 1139.

Boden SD et al. "Abnormal magnetic-resonance scans of the lumbar spine in asymptomatic subjects: A prospective investigation." *Journal of Bone and Joint Surgery* (1990); 72: 403 - 8.

Kobayashi, K et al. "Complications associated with spine surgery in patients aged 80 years or older: Japan Association of Spine Surgeons with Ambition (JASA) multicenter study." *Global Spine Journal* (2017); 7: 636 - 641.

Martin, BI et al. "Trends in Lumbar Fusion Procedure Rates and Associated Hospital Costs for Degenerative Spinal Diseases in the United States, 2004 to 2015." *Spine* (2019); 44: 369 - 376.

Nguyen, TH et al. "Long-term outcomes of lumbar fusion among worker's compensation subjects." *Spine* (2010); 20: 1 - 11.

Schug, SA and EM Pogatzki-Zahn. "Chronic pain after surgery or injury." *Pain: Clinical Updates. International Association for the Study of Pain* (2011); 19: 1 - 5.

Young, AK et al. "Assessment of presurgical psychological screening in patients undergoing spine surgery." *Journal of Spinal Disorders and Techniques* (2014); 27: 76 - 79.

Chapter 9

Boden SD et al. "Abnormal magnetic-resonance scans of the lumbar spine in asymptomatic subjects: A prospective investigation." *Journal of Bone and Joint Surgery* (1990); 72: 403 - 8.

Brox, JI et al. "Randomized clinical trial of lumbar instrumented fusion and cognitive intervention and exercises in patients with chronic low back pain and disc degeneration." *Spine* (2003); 28(17): 1913 - 1921.

Brox, JI et al. "Lumbar instrumented fusion compared with cognitive intervention and exercises in patients with chronic back pain after previous surgery for disc herniation: A prospective randomized controlled study." *Pain* (2006); 122: 145 - 55.

Carragee EJ, et al. "A Gold Standard Evaluation of the 'Discogenic Pain' Diagnosis as Determined by Provocative Discography." *Spine* (2006) 31: 2115 - 2123.

Fairbanks, J et al. "Randomized controlled trial to compare surgical stabilization of the lumbar spine with an intensive rehabilitation program for patients with chronic low back pain: the MRC spine stabilization trial." *BMJ* (2005); doi:L10:10.1136/bmj.38441.BF.

Franklin, GM et al. "Outcome of lumbar fusion in Washington State Workers' Compensation." *Spine* (1994); 19: 1897 - 1903.

Fritzell, P. et al. "Cost-effectiveness of lumbar fusion and nonsurgical treatment for chronic low back pain in the Swedish Lumbar Spine Study: A multicenter, randomized, controlled trial from the Swedish Lumbar Spine Study Group." *Spine* (2004); 29: 421 - 34; discussion Z3.

Hashmi, JA et al. "Shape shifting pain: Chronification of back pain shifts brain representation from nociceptive to emotional circuits." *Brain* (2013); 136: 2751 - 2768.

Giesecke, T et al. "Evidence of augmented central pain processing in idiopathic chronic low back pain." *Arthritis and Rheumatism* (2004); 50: 613 - 623.

Jarvik, JG et al. "Three-year incidence of low back pain in an initially asymptomatic cohort: Clinical and imaging risk factors." *Spine* (2005); 30: 1541 - 1548.

Kerezoudis, P et al. "Returns to the operating room after neurosurgical procedures in a tertiary care academic medical center: Implications for health care policy and quality improvement." Neurosurgery (2018); 0: 1 - 10.

Martin, BI et al. "Trends in Lumbar Fusion Procedure Rates and Associated Hospital Costs for Degenerative Spinal Diseases in the United States, 2004 to 2015." Spine (2019); 44: 369 - 376.

Mooney, V. "Point of View." Spine (2001); 26: 2532 - 2533.

Nguyen, TH et al. "Long-term outcomes of lumbar fusion among worker's compensation subjects." Spine (2010); 20: 1 - 11.

Perkins, FM and H Kehlet. "Chronic pain as an outcome of surgery: A Review of Predictive Factors." Anesthesiology (2000); 93: 1123 - 1133.

Schug, SA and EM Pogatzki-Zahn. "Chronic pain after surgery or injury." Pain: Clinical Updates. International Association for the Study of Pain (2011); 19: 1 - 5.

Sham, Maghout-Juratli G et al. "Lumbar fusion outcomes in Washington State Worker's Compensation." Spine (2006); 23: 2715 - 23.

Young, AK et al. "Assessment of presurgical psychological screening in patients undergoing spine surgery." *Journal of Spinal Disorders and Techniques* (2014); 27: 76 - 79.

Appendix A

Boden SD, et al. "Abnormal magnetic-resonance scans of the lumbar spine in asymptomatic subjects: A prospective investigation." *Journal of Bone and Joint Surgery* (1990); 72: 403 - 8.

Jarvik, JG et al. "Three-year incidence of low back pain in an initially asymptomatic cohort: Clinical and imaging risk factors." *Spine* (2005); 30: 1541 - 1548.

Goz et al. "Perioperative complications and mortality after spinal fusions." *Spine* (2013); 38(22): 1970 - 1976

Hashmi, JA et al. "Shape shifting pain: chronification of back pain shifts brain representation from nociceptive to emotional circuits." *Brain* (2013); 136: 2751 - 2768.

Herno, A et al. "The long-term prognosis after operation for lumbar spinal stenosis." *Scandinavian Journal of Rehabilitation Medicine* (1993); 25: 167–71.

Martin, BI et al. "Trends in Lumbar Fusion Procedure Rates and Associated Hospital Costs for Degenerative Spinal Diseases in the United States, 2004 to 2015." *Spine* (2019); 44: 369 - 376.

Nachemson, AF et al. "Intravital dynamic pressure measurements in lumbar discs: A study of common movements, maneuvers, and exercises." *Scandinavian Journal of Rehabilitation Medicine Supplement* (1970); 1: 1 - 40.

Nachemson, AF. "The lumbar spine: An orthopedic challenge." *Spine* (1976); 1: 59 - 71.

Nachemson, AF. "Adult scoliosis and back pain." Spine (1979); 4: 513 - 517.

Ribeiro, RP et al. "Spontaneous regression of symptomatic lumbar disc herniation." Acta Reumatol Port. (2011); 36: 396 - 8.

Shan, Z, et al. Spontaneous Resorption of lumbar disc herniation is less likely with Modic changes are present. Spine (2014); 39:736 - 744.

Weber, H. Lumbar disc herniation: A controlled, prospective study with ten years of observation. Spine (1983); 8:131 - 140.

Appendix B

Carragee, EJ, et al. "A prospective controlled study of limited versus subtotal posterior discectomy: Short-term outcomes in patients with herniated lumbar intervertebral discs and large posterior annular defect." *Spine* (2006); 31: 653 - 657.

Daubs, MD et al. "Does correction of preoperative coronal imbalance make a difference in outcomes of adult patients with deformity?" *Spine* (2013; 38: 476 - 483.

Frymoyer, JW et al. "A comparison of radiographic findings in fusion and non-fusion patients ten or more years following lumbar disc surgery." *Spine* (1979); 5: 435 - 440.

Hashmi, JA et al. "Shape shifting pain: Chronification of back pain shifts brain representation from nociceptive to emotional circuits." *Brain* (2013); 136: 2751 - 2768.

Herno, A et al. "The long-term prognosis after operation for lumbar spinal stenosis." Scandinavian Journal of Rehabilitation Medicine (1993); 25: 167–71.

Kelly, MP et al. "Operative versus non-operative treatment for adult symptomatic scoliosis." *Journal of Bone and Joint Surgery* (2019); 101: 338 - 352.

Kim, JK et al. "Proximal junctional kyphosis in adult spinal deformity after segmental posterior spinal instrumentation and fusion." *Spine* (2008); 33: 2179 - 2184.

Lehr, MA et al. "Patients cannot reliably distinguish the iliac crest bone graft donor site from the contralateral side after lumbar spine fusion." *Spine* (2018); 44; 527 - 533.

Martin, BI et al. "Reoperation rates following lumbar spine surgery and the influence of spinal fusion procedures." *Spine* (2007); 32: 382 - 387.

Martin, BI et al. "Trends in Lumbar Fusion Procedure Rates and Associated Hospital Costs for Degenerative Spinal Diseases in the United States, 2004 to 2015." *Spine* (2019); 44: 369 - 376.

Pitter, FT et al. "Revision risk after primary adult spinal deformity surgery: A nationwide study with two-year follow-up." Spine Deformity (2019); 20: 619-626.

INDEX

rewiring of, 80–81
Brox, J. I., 123–124
bulging discs, 140, 190–193
bureaucracy, dealing with, 42
burning sensation, 31, 144, 147,
149

cadaver bone, 198
cages, spinal, 122, 206–207
calcium, 165
calm nervous systems, 5, 36. *See
also* nervous system status;
*specific conditions and
procedures*
cancer, 20, 27–28. *See also*
tumors
cardiopulmonary failure, 173–
174
carpal tunnel syndrome (CTS),
148
Carragee, Eugene, 118–120
cauda equina, 184
cauda equina syndrome, 31–34,
144, 190
central nervous system (CNS),
35, 184
central stenosis, 23
cerebrospinal fluid (CSF), 188
cervical stenosis, 147
change, resistance to, 48
chondromalacia of the patella,
27, 143–144
chronic pain
overview of, 63–64, 75
defined, 63
evolution of, 67–74
memorization of, 4, 22, 48,
67–70, 117
modifiers of, 70–74, 77–78
nervous system status and,
64–67
sensitization to, 67–68
as surgical complication, 8,

118
*See also specific conditions and
procedures*
chronic pain resolution
action steps, 81–88
anxiety and, 77–78
benefits of, 93
prehab and, 89–92
principles of, 78–81
taking charge of own care and,
85–88
chronic stress, 38–40
circumferential fusion, 197
CNS (central nervous system),
35, 184
cognitive-perceptual disruption,
45
collapsing scoliosis, 174
collapsing spinal deformity, 16
compensated deformity, 160–
161
complications
chronic pain and, 8, 118
Fritzell study and, 128
fusions, 118
location and, 184
major versus minor, 102–104
risk-benefit surgery analysis
and, 8
screw placement problems,
159
spinal deformity surgery,
221–222
*See also specific conditions and
procedures*
compression, 15, 23–25. *See also*
decompression procedures
compression fractures, 177–181,
216–217
congenital indifference to pain,
65
congenital spinal stenosis, 148
congenital spondylolisthesis, 151